D1083400

But You
Look
So Well

But You Look So Well

John R. Ginther

Nelson Hall *nh* Chicago

Excerpt from "Reason for Music" (p. 67). Copyright© 1972
by Archibald MacLeish. Reprinted by permission of Houghton
Mifflin Company.

LIBRARY OF CONGRESS CATALOGING IN PUBLICATION DATA

Ginther, John Robert, 1922–
    But you look so well.

    1.   Multiple sclerosis—Biography.   2.   Ginther,
John Robert, 1922–   I.   Title.
RC377.G56   616.8′34′00926   77–26009
ISBN 0–88229–399–0

Manufactured in the United States of America

10   9   8   7   6   5   4   3   2   1

Contents

Preface

In the course of events in our life my wife, Kay, and I found ourselves in a discussion group with other couples, each of which had one spouse afflicted with multiple sclerosis. We chatted, expounded, and discussed symptoms, feelings, beliefs, and frustrations. At one point Dr. Marcia Pavlou, one of the psychologists in attendance, asked whether I had ever thought of writing about my recollections of the course of my multiple sclerosis. I do not recall my exact response to her, but the question became a challenge. This short work is the result. I saw her at the time of my clinic appointment in February of 1975, a few months after the challenge. It was then she learned that a book had been written. When she asked what plans there were for the manuscript, I replied that perhaps others might benefit from reading it. She said she believed that indeed others might learn from it. If Ms. Pavlou is correct, I would be thankful.

The information and incidents related in this book, except those which are autobiographical, are from a number of sources. Books containing research reports about multiple sclerosis and the general class of demyelinating diseases yielded most of the technical information. Neurology textbooks also were helpful. Papers from a symposium at the 1974 meeting of the American Psychological Association in New Orleans are discussed in Chapter VIII. That symposium was entitled "Psychology and Health: Clinical Psychological Services to Multiple Sclerosis Patients." Michael F. Hartings, Ph.D., of the Multiple Sclerosis Center at Rush-Presbyterian-St. Luke's Hospital in Chicago, organized the symposium and was its chairman. Papers presented and their authors were: "A Neurologist's Perspective on Multiple Sclerosis," Floyd A. Davis, M.D., director of the Multiple Sclerosis Center at Rush; "Cognitive, Emotional, and Personality Correlates of Multiple Sclerosis," Susan L. Andrews, Ph.D., associate professor of psychology, University of Wisconsin-Waukesha County, Waukesha, Wisconsin; "A Program of Comprehensive Health Care for the Multiple Sclerosis Patient," Marcia M. Pavlou, M.A. (now Ph.D.), program coordinator, Multiple Sclerosis Center at Rush; "Community Mental Health Services and Multiple Sclerosis," William B. Cammin, Ph.D., program director, Bay-Arenac Community Mental Health Board, Bay City, Michigan; and "Group Psychotherapy with Multiple Sclerosis Patients and Their Spouses," Melvin L. Schwartz, Ph.D., Wayne State University School of Medicine, Detroit, Michigan. Although I have not read the last paper, an overview of it was included in the prospectus which accompanies the symposium proposal.

Informal situations which contributed to the book include three sessions of a week each with patients at the camp sponsored annually by the Chicago Chapter of the National Multiple Sclerosis Society, a series of discussions in a group at the Rush-Presbyterian-St. Luke's Multiple Sclerosis Center, and informal chats with friends and acquaintances who either are afflicted with multiple sclerosis or have a friend so afflicted. Also contributing to my experiences were discussions with eight physicians, three of whom were neurologists.

The interaction in my mind of the thoughts and ideas from these people, events, books and documents resulted in this autobiographical primer on multiple sclerosis.

When first this episode in our lives was recorded, the writing was guided by my vivid recollection of events and my subjective interrelating of them. One result, it seemed, was a vagueness, a haziness about time and the sequence of events. After the fact, and in light of a suggestion, a new opening chapter was developed. It contains the time line for events taken directly from my physician's oral report of my records.

Preceding the chronology in the new opening chapter are my purposes for writing the manuscript. Next some explanation is offered of the forces which impinged on our decisions and actions; decisions and actions which may seem odd to the reader, but which seemed natural to us during the long years spent struggling with multiple sclerosis.

Then we come to the chronology which leads directly to the physician's disclosure of the diagnosis to me, the opening event in the second chapter.

1
Why?

To be stricken by a dread disease is a frightening experience. To successfully ward off or to recover from some of the major symptoms is a religious experience. It has been our lot to endure the former and enjoy the latter during the episode in which I was stricken with multiple sclerosis. But of the three of us I alone was to live in ignorance of the diagnosis for many years, and that is a damning experience. Unfortunately, Kay and our daughter, Diane, matched my unique experience with their psychological agony as they observed me and heeded the physician's advice to withhold the diagnosis from me.

At the suggestion of a professional psychologist who deals constantly with multiple sclerosis patients, I have prepared this report of the events in this episode of our lives. Perhaps it will offer hope to many newly stricken and their families. My avowed intentions, however, are different from offering hope. The first purpose is to acquaint the reader with the basic nature of the disease as well as the symptoms and the diagnostic procedures often used to identify it. The second purpose is to point out from personal experience the psychological involvement which accompanies the symptoms.

The physician informed my family of the diagnosis soon after it had been confirmed by a neurologist in 1962 and, as you shall see, recommended against informing me. When you learn that I remained ignorant of the diagnosis until May of 1971, you may properly ask why. Why did I not ask more questions about the events during the ten-year span after the diagnosis, or in the years which preceded the diagnosis? In retrospect one might change the question and inquire about the circumstances in which a patient could permit a physician to refrain from saying more than he did about the ailments which beset this patient. The answers are not easy to recall, but perhaps an attempt at reconstruction would be useful.

First it must be said that we had confidence in our physician. This confidence had at least three bases. For one thing a large number of our friends and acquaintances used his service. This circle of persons, although perhaps not unique, included many extraordinary individuals: some were members of families of faculty from The University of Chicago; all were from the Hyde Park neighborhood. A mystique prevailed akin to that in colleges which assign a student to his graduating class when first he matriculates. That remains his class no matter the intervening difficulties which may arise in that student's studies or life. In our neighborhood your physician, no matter the minor problems or irritations which arose with his care, was your physician. At one time or another he no doubt had attended the neighborhood university. Some member of either his or his wife's family was no doubt an old-timer in the Hyde Park community. With reasons such as these, who would dare lack confidence in his physician?

But if local factors seem insufficient to generate confidence, one needs but be reminded of the almost reverent attitude toward physicians which historically permeated the populace and still is noticeable in the conversations of many patients. Skillful use of mass media by interested parties played some part in developing this attitude. For example, no matter the drug or remedy being advertised, the listener was admonished to "see your doctor." And the growing shortage of physicians sprang, it was well known, from the extraordinary efforts of the American Medical Association to keep medical standards high. If you did not have confidence in your physician, perhaps you were also un-American.

In our case a third base for confidence was the care we had received and continued to receive. A spectacular example is the fact that Kay's left hand functions as well as ever following a kitchen accident which could have ended her hobby of playing the organ. One can hardly find a scar from either the operation or the wound, a puncture by a sliver of glass which severed the tendon to her small finger, rendering it unusable. Our physician, who had trained as a surgeon while practicing family medicine, was himself rather pleased with the repair work.

Confidence in our physician is but one of the complex reasons which perhaps explain, or suggest, why I did not raise more questions about what was happening to me. A second possible reason is the nature of the medical events which I endured. Each seemed self-contained. Each of the major apparent problems either turned out to be a false alarm—the possible heart attack—or seemed to have been overcome in short order—a gall bladder attack and a vision problem. This point is made again later and explored in some detail.

Why did Kay not tell me the secret? Why did she remain silent for a decade? The reasons parallel those which have already been suggested as reasons for my not pressing to learn more about what was happening. She had confidence in the physician as did I.

No doubt the early years of silence stemmed primarily from fear. Nevertheless, it must have been confidence in the physician which led her to accept his reason for withholding the secret from me. Kay recalls that he said something like: "Look! He's a busy man and he has a responsible position. He doesn't need to be bothered with concern about this for the time being. If I can give him one year, or one month without worrying about this I will think I have done a good thing. Don't you agree?"

If that seemed an appropriate reason to the physician it should be, and was, reason enough for the patient's family. Furthermore, one can hardly disagree with anyone who is acting with such moral purpose. When later he restored function in her finger, confidence was reinforced.

The matrix, or perhaps that is too neat a concept—the slough of impressions, reasons, attitudes, fears, and other feelings through which a path of action was being felt, one cautious step at a time, does not permit a precise description of the path. Kay's influence on me, following the lead of our physician, helped lull me into a state of naive though hardly blissful acceptance of the day by day situation. Reinforcement of my confidence in the physician developed on the morning he telephoned from the operating suite to inform me that the pathologist's report indicated that Kay had cancer. He said a radical mastectomy was indicated, and asked my thoughts on the matter. I of course consented and thanked him for calling. This kind of partnership in a major decision no doubt added to the unfathomable morass out of which my continuing almost unquestioning faith arose about my own situation. Perhaps I never entertained the possibility of deviousness on his part, with regard to my condition.

Of course the mind-boggling realization that my wife,

Diane's mother, had been struck by the dreaded killer cancer served to shift the focus of thoughts away from me for many months. I borrowed Diane's bicycle to ride the mile-and-a-half round trip to the hospital twice daily. At first there was great need for buoying Kay's spirit above the depths of despair, distracting her mind from the torturing pain, and curbing her imagination from the inevitable projections involving disfigurement and womanliness. After several weeks these many needs were partially replaced by the restrained joy of visiting a drive-in daily for a chocolate malted milk to help restore some of Kay's lost nutrients and weight. Thus for perhaps months there was little time and no emotional space for concern about my relatively minor problems.

The knot of questions about why the physician withheld the diagnosis from the patient, why the patient progressed so far into the syndrome of symptoms without pressing for more information, and why the patient's wife permitted these situations to continue is difficult to answer. Perhaps it is clear that the answers are by no means certain; that they have an indistinctness perhaps analogous to French impressionistic art. I have tried to establish, in retrospect, what may be warrantable assertions about the matters.

That I am less than happy about the physician's initial decision to withhold the diagnosis from me should be abundantly clear from a reading of Chapter 3. It is perhaps significant that after patronizing this physician over a period of twenty-six years, the last sixteen of which constituted a continuous period of family care, we no longer seek his services or counsel. Toward the end we drifted apart, with apparent mutual awareness and consent. The drift began at about the time I informed Kay of my problem and learned that for years she had been privy to the diagnosis. Recently someone suggested that the physician had engaged "in some curious behavior to say the least." No doubt others will agree.

Earlier I suggested that the initial years of Kay's silence, her willingness to carry the burden of the diagnosis without disclosing it to me, may have stemmed from fear. The attitude of the physician, suggesting that the patient was being spared an awful truth, no doubt contributed to that fear. Also, dealing with the unknown or the misunderstood can induce and cultivate fear. That she was attempting to cope by becoming informed is clear from Kay's tale of contacting the Chicago Chapter of the National Multiple Sclerosis Society. She sought information, and felt that this organization might be able to furnish some. This, one should note, happened in the early 1960's.

She found the address of the local chapter in the telephone book and paid a visit to the address on Michigan Avenue in Chicago. It was, she relates, a small, one-room office with one lady working, apparently as a one-woman office. Literature was stacked in slight disarray all around on the floor and on the sparse furniture. It was apparently a scene reflecting pitifully deep poverty, a scene perhaps too often repeated in social agencies.

Such a depressing scene only enlarges the sphere of fear. But the tragic blow came from the literature itself. Consider the following contemporary magazine advertisement by the National Multiple Sclerosis Society: "Multiple Sclerosis cripples young adults. We don't want your sympathy. We just want your help. We can win this one." It is frighteningly informative yet it contains a confident note of hope. Contrast this with the following information offered in medical sources of the late fifties and early sixties: multiple sclerosis is a progressively worsening disease with no known cure. This, in fact, was what the lady in the office of the Chicago Chapter of the National Multiple Sclerosis Society said to Kay. The effect must have been about the same as that of catching an unexpectedly heavy medicine ball in the belly. Kay says that the literature carried information with the same basic message. I have been unable to locate copies of the literature distributed by the MS Society at the time, but examination of sources of information, that is medical texts, etc., support Kay's contention. In addition to the statement above about "a progressively worsening disease" the literature carried other hope-inspiring messages such as "if you have the disease you may expect always to have it" and "it may cripple you but very likely you will not die from it." As early as 1961, however, there also appeared in medical literature statements suggesting that there were various degrees of severity to attacks of multiple sclerosis, suggesting also that there were degrees of recovery possible. These latter statements seem to have been overlooked by persons in agencies to which families turned for hope.

It is easy for me to believe and to understand that my wife was filled with fear, that she was ready to accept the physician's suggestion that the patient not be told. What could she tell me? Perhaps that I was becoming a hopeless cripple? That she was prepared to abandon her accustomed roles and become the breadwinner? Fear unquestionably joined forces with confidence in the physician to lead Kay to burden herself with the secret, thus attempting to shield me. One of the subsequent events of our life, her radical mastectomy, we believe to have been, to a significant degree, a consequence of the extended period of distress she endured under the burden of silence about my condition.

In retrospect one can imagine that these three forces, confidence in the physician, the nature of the symptomatic episodes, and fear, combined to cause our behavior: Kay's withholding the diagnosis from me, and my continued acceptance of the minuscule amounts of information offered by the physician.

The process of recalling and reporting my experiences

with multiple sclerosis could leave the reader bewildered about the time element and chronology of events. This is the case in part because I did not have access to the files in which the dates of the events are recorded until after the manuscript was completed.

But there is another possible reason for time distortion. Consider the following categories of events for ailments: initial attacks, duration of condition, and exacerbations and remissions. These categories yield information which differs widely in the case of multiple sclerosis from that for more common diseases or conditions. Sprains, cuts and bruises, colds, measles, influenza, appendectomies— such aggravations last a few days. They become concerns if not cleared away in less than a week or ten days. With the symptoms of multiple sclerosis, however, one strives to learn to measure, endure, and anticipate in periods of months and years. This may be one basis for a distorted sense of time. Attacks seem interminable because they may last for months rather than days. Mix a conventional, habitual time unit of a week together with an enforced time unit of months, with some symptoms enduring for years, and some time disorientation may be expected to result.

With the hope that inclusion of an accurate chronology would be helpful, one has been included at this point. I was surprised to learn that several events took place within a period of thirteen months between October of 1961 and November of 1962. It was illuminating to notice the long spans of time some of the symptoms endured; for example double vision was noted by the physician in April of 1962 and in May of 1970. It persists to this day in events which are reported later. The dates and events listed here were reported to me over the telephone by the physician as he scanned my file in October 1976.

The fateful day was March 27, 1959, although I am uncertain whether this was the day a sebacious cyst was removed or whether this was four days afterward, the day I reported numbness in my hand and finger. But March 27, 1959 is the initial entry in this chronology. The next entry is October 1961 when I was hospitalized with chest pains and examined thoroughly by a cardiologist. In December 1961 I reported having numbness in the right hip and leg, numbness which began during a trip to Cleveland. In January 1962 came another hospitalization to enable a myelogram to be taken. In April 1962 double vision occurred. At that time referral was made to both an ophthalmologist and a neurologist. It was then that the suspected diagnosis was confirmed, although I could only guess at this fact when writing about the referrals. This was also probably the time at which Kay and Diane were informed of the diagnosis. During November 1962 came another hospitalization for observation for a suspected gall bladder problem. In June 1963 the files indicate that my reflexes were normal but in December of the same year there was numbness in the lower rim of the pelvis. Observation continued until May 1965 when hypersensitivity of the left side of the head and ear were placed in the record.

Bear in mind that this chronology is not a complete listing of my appointments with the physician. Rather it is his indication of the onset of notable symptoms or changes in symptoms. Three years elapsed before the next problem arose. In May 1968 I reported in with hypersensitivity of the left foot and jerking of the leg at night. From this point forward hypersensitivity of one or both feet never disappeared, and leg jerks, both right and left were almost nightly occurrences. The physician's report failed to indicate the date of onset of numbness in both legs. It probably began in the next onslaught.

After the appearance of no new symptoms for nearly two years, the record for May 1970 indicates that I had begun having balance problems. In July of the same year my right ear began itching. This problem was to intensify and last into 1974. In July 1970 and again in November 1970 I was referred to an ear specialist for advice on the continuing problem. In May 1971 an acute bladder problem resulted in treatment in the emergency room of the hospital in my home town, Sturgis, Michigan. Upon release by the local physician I promised and did go immediately to my regular physician. Within the next few days he became convinced that he should disclose the suspected diagnosis to me. This was twelve years after the first apparent symptom came to his attention.

In August 1971 the record indicates "unsteadiness." In November 1971 I sought advice about the right ear from another specialist. At the August 1972 appointment with my regular physician I indicated fatigue. A year later, in August 1973, the report indicates "run-down; neurologic signs negative." In December 1973 the neurologist to whom I had been referred reconfirmed the diagnosis, indicating the condition was benign. June 1974 marked my last visit to our physician; no doubt it was for my annual physical examination. Except for the October telephone call, my last conversation with him was in September 1976. He asked how I was getting along and I congratulated him on his accurate diagnosis of my elusive problems.

My subsequent medical advice has come from a medical center which specializes in multiple sclerosis. My health, outside the myriad neurologically based difficulties, has always been excellent. A tonsillectomy in elementary school years and an appendectomy during my twenties are the most serious health problems I have had.

2
What Is MS?

At one point during the dozen years before my physician let me in on the secret, I recall saying to him: "Maybe some day I'll ask you what the problem is." His reply was: "Maybe I'll tell you." The matter was pressed no further. But years later, after an incident which is reported in Chapter 5, he finally sat down and said: "Maybe it's time to tell you." After a pause he continued: "This may come as a shock to you. For a number of years we have suspected that you had multiple sclerosis." During the ensuing silence I was not shocked; puzzled is perhaps a more accurate description, for I had no earthly idea what multiple sclerosis was. It is not at all certain that I had ever heard the term previously. Except for my hastily forming plans to read about multiple sclerosis, nothing more comes to mind about this visit to the physician's office.

Upon emerging from the clinic my steps must have headed directly to the library in Billings Hospital on the campus of The University of Chicago. There was some kind of construction being done which necessitated that the library be housed in a different place in the medical school. I found my way there and examined the card catalogue, which led me to a section of the stacks which housed books on neurology. There I found what proved to be the only non-technical book on the topic in the Billings Library. The table of contents listed a number of personally familiar subjects suggesting some of the difficulties which had mysteriously beset me over the past dozen years. Although it is certain that I turned hurriedly to the chapter which held promise of defining or describing the disease, it is equally certain that the quick perusal of the contents stirred many memories. Topics such as jerking, dizziness, fatigue, bowel function, operations and anesthesia, and bladder all touched off reconstructions from memory of unpleasant incidents heretofore unrelated in my mind.

The chapter telling about the disease was interesting although distressing. An early assertion was that the cause of multiple sclerosis was unknown. A quick look at the date of copyright, a decade earlier, provided dim hope that the book was out of date on this topic. The further assertion that a cure was not known was disheartening although not altogether surprising. Before arriving at a descriptive statement of the disease I also discovered that the disease may cripple you. After having spent twelve years enduring one symptom after another, faithfully reporting to my physician, making the rounds of several specialists, finally being told what the name of the condition was, and reading a table of contents, an entire short chapter, and more than a single paragraph in the chapter most narrowly focused on the disease, I still didn't know much about MS.

Finally, this statement appeared: "Multiple sclerosis damages the nerve coverings." My education had begun. Although much that was to be read later would be technical, my first encounter with a book about multiple sclerosis was noticeably laced with suggestions that one should accept himself as disabled. Not that one should despair; rather, the great powers of recuperation and compensation were important assets to the disabled. A listing of types of effectively functioning people included the blind, those without stomachs, and so on. The shock that my physician had mentioned now struck. An entire half day was consumed in reading and scanning the neurology section of the stacks. It was disquieting to notice books on psychiatry close at hand while scanning the neurology section.

My search extended into the periodical literature even that first day, as I discovered what motivation to read really enables one to do. Slowly the nature of multiple sclerosis was revealed as a condition in which the myelin, that is the fatty sheath which surrounds nerve fibers, is destroyed and replaced by scar tissue. It occurred to me that this was somewhat like stripping insulation off electrical wires, then wrapping them with metal foil. Some short-circuiting seems inevitable. In the case of the nerve fibers, they seem destined to be excited inadvertently by the scar tissue. These two possibilities would account for several symptomatic conditions: unsteadiness, bumping, and other conditions caused by failure of a message to get through, and uncontrollable jerkings, itchings, nervous discomfort, and other symptoms apparently resulting from excitation by scar tissue.

Having discovered that the nerve sheath, called myelin, was involved in the disease, I felt it necessary to learn more about myelin. Efforts to do this stretched over a period of three years. The search was fruitful even if the terminology encountered was bewildering at times for a layman. In research papers and in summaries of research there seemed to be some agreement on the value of myelin, that is in terms of its usefulness. For example, in one book purporting to summarize biochemical findings, one finds the statement that the only known function of myelin is the assistance of propagation of the nerve impulse. I assume that an appropriate synonym for "propagate" is "transmit" or "conduct." Myelin, as we shall see later, is wrapped in layers around a nerve fiber. Research asserts that fibers with more layers of myelin conduct more rapidly than do fibers with fewer layers.

In another book, focusing on studies of myelin, its development and destruction, is found the statement that the main role of myelin is to act as insulation, apparently so nerve impulses will stay on the right wire, so to speak. If you examine an enlarged picture of a cross section of a bundle of nerve fibers, it looks a little like the opened top of a package of cigarettes. Myelin seems to remind you of the paper wrapping of each of the cigarettes. However, myelin seems seldom to occur as a single-layered cover. Rather, it is wrapped around each nerve several times. The central nervous system is reported never to be covered as heavily, that is with as many wrappings of myelin, as is the peripheral system. In animals the difference in number of wrappings ranges from around a dozen to as many as a hundred on a single nerve fiber.

One more observation concerning myelin may suggest its delicate nature, if thinness is a criterion for or a characteristic of delicateness. Returning to the image of the opened package of cigarettes, the cross section of nerve fibers, when magnified 44,000 times, appears to be about the size of cigarettes, perhaps ranging up to the diameter of a fat cigar. The myelin is only the outer sheath for the nerve and, when magnified as described, each layer of wrapping appears to be no thicker than a line drawn with the point of a fairly well-sharpened pencil. Dividing the thickness of the line into quarters would still leave you with a magnification factor of about 10,000. One wonders how so much of our nervous system remains intact and operative, and what the potential of the human would be if he were completely free from the microscopic internal injuries to the nerves which must affect us all in one way or another.

Myelin has yet another characteristic: it is said to be stable. The meaning here is apparently based on metabolic turnover, that is how rapidly the substance is changed into something else and replaced. Lipid, a fat which is insoluble in water, and protein are known ingredients of myelin. Both lipids and proteins are used and replaced everywhere in the human body. To say that myelin is stable in the metabolic sense means that the lipid and protein factors are not typically used and replenished as they are in other storehouses of the body. In fact, myelin, it is said, cannot easily be drawn upon to feed the metabolic process. The consequences of this assertion can be seen in studies of adult rats in which the brain suffered very little, if any, in states of severe undernutrition even though much of the brain weight is attributable to myelin, which theoretically could have been used to alleviate the state of metabolic hunger.

My wanderings through textbooks and research reports dealing with multiple sclerosis revealed that a great deal was known about the condition, but very little of the information was of use to the patient. For example, some slowing of the flow of blood to cells in the central nervous system seems to occur in the disease. A variety of methods for increasing the blood flow have been tried. This approach to alleviating a symptom has now fallen from favor. It is known that saturated fats tend to clog blood vessels, restricting the flow of blood. At one time this suggested the possibility that improper diet might be the cause of multiple sclerosis. However the theorists on nutrition constructed the logic, a large-scale research effort was mounted to attempt to prevent, stop, perhaps even reverse the course of multiple sclerosis through the manipulation of diet. This avenue, as so many others, fell short of the goal.

Among the promising conceptions of the cause of multiple sclerosis, two seem to be the most prominent in the minds of present-day investigators. The first of these hypotheses is that a virus is the agent. The second suggests that an autoimmune mechanism is at work. This means a rejection of part of your own tissue by your normally helpful protective agents or mechanisms. It is even thought possible that both these hypothetical causes can be entertained in the same theory. This would mean that some virus would invade the body and act upon something (white blood cells seem to be involved) which triggers an autoimmune reaction, which then destroys tissue.

Before persuing autoimmune reaction let me digress a moment to indicate a vague parallel between the "incubation" periods for multiple sclerosis and some forms of cancer. Just reported above is the theory that a virus invades and acts upon the system to trigger the autoimmune reaction. But the time interval between the invasion and the appearance of symptoms of multiple sclerosis is thought to be several years in length. In some forms of cancer, it is believed, a cell must mutate four or five times, over a period of perhaps fifteen years, before dividing and growing out of control. (Since most cells do not live that many years, what is meant seems to be that the line or descendants of the mutant cell mutate again and again until the cancer begins.) The mutants in the development of many forms of cancer are, very likely, agents in the environment, carcinogens. Many people are not convinced that reduction of this or that carcinogen is desirable or necessary if the incidence of cancer is to be reduced. In large part, no doubt, this reluctance to accept the fact of carcinogens is due to the time lag for effects, the time necessary for several mutations to occur before a cell becomes cancerous.

The "incubation" period, then, is lengthy for both multiple sclerosis and cancer. In the case of some types of cancer a substantial theory is offered to explain or account for the time. A similar explanatory theory seems missing for multiple sclerosis.

Multiple sclerosis is but one of a dozen or more clinical conditions which are hypothesized to result from some kind or form of autoimmune action. By now everyone is familiar with the problems of tissue rejection encountered in organ transplants. In the case of a transplant, the body's mechanism recognizes the new organ as foreign, and attacks it to rid the body of it. (Whether the mechanism recognizes the tissue as foreign or fails to recognize it as acceptable is a matter which may be very important to researchers on the topic, but we more or less equate the two possibilities here.) In the case of MS, the mechanism somehow suddenly fails to recognize its own myelin, and destroys it. Later in this chapter several types or degrees of MS are suggested. Depending upon the type of MS, myelin may be destroyed in almost insignificant amounts, or in amounts and places sufficient to lead to clear symptoms of varying degrees of severity, or in such quantity that the nervous system becomes so unreliable that survival is no longer possible.

It is said that many of the diseases or clinical conditions involving an autoimmune mechanism result from another kind of mechanism known as an auto-sensitization mechanism. Auto-sensitization is linked with hypersensitivity by some researchers, but this hypersensitivity is a condition different from the hypersensitivity reported as prevalent among MS patients. It is thought that a delayed-type hypersensitivity of the first kind might have a major role in autoimmune diseases like MS. The second type of hypersensitivity is that which seems to require scratching or rubbing. Having said a bit about autoimmune conditions, let us now turn to conditions in which myelin is destroyed, for they are not always the same as the autoimmune conditions.

First, perhaps a few words about the usual locations of myelin destruction are in order. Typically, damage to the nerve covering is restricted to three specific areas of the central nervous system in multiple sclerosis. Lesions in the spinal column are responsible for symptoms almost too numerous to list. A partial recitation includes paralysis in one or more limbs, absence of sensations, lack of position sense, bladder and bowel dysfunctions, unsteady gait, numbness, stumbling, and weakness in an extremity. All symptoms, including retention and incontinence in bladder and bowel functions may come and go without apparent cause. Lesions on the brain stem may result in a variety of visual problems including blurred and double vision as well as slurred speech. Attacks on the cerebrum affect thinking and orientation. It is believed that such attacks appear later than attacks on the spinal column. This list foreshadows much of my story.

It is known that there are several conditions in which myelin is destroyed. Among those listed are some virus infections and, incidentally, carbon monoxide poisoning. Two well-known students of MS whom I have heard speak both stated that a virus is involved and that, furthermore, this invasion probably occurs before you enter the teens. Whatever action this virus takes, the consequences often are not apparent for many years. Whether it lies dormant before acting, something analogous to the seventeen-year locust, or whether the condition it establishes simply lurks about awaiting appropriate circumstances before striking is not clear.

Eventually all investigative roads, at least those about MS, lead to biochemistry. Among the objects studied by biochemists are antibodies. Several of these antibodies act on particular components of the central nervous system, the site of demyelination in MS. More specifically, certain antibodies in nerve tissue have an effect which results in demyelination. Such antibodies have been found in fluids from patients with MS, particularly, it seems, in the cerebrospinal fluid.

Of special interest to me, though not directly relevant to my case, is the likelihood that malnutrition or undernourishment may cause a deficiency in myelination. It is known that intellectual development can be impaired by undernourishment, and it is known that the myelin sheath is capable of playing a part in the activities of the central nervous system. Recall, for example, that the thickness of the sheath is directly related to speed of transmission along a nerve. So perhaps the specter of the unsheathed nerve should replace that of the bloated belly when we think of undernourished children; a bloated belly can often be overcome but a deficiency in intellectual development stemming from a lack of myelin sheathing may be irreparable.

One of the primary reasons for the primitive state of knowledge about the causes of MS is that it is so difficult to study in the human. Even if biochemical investigations of myelination and demyelination in live humans were attempted, the results would not be attainable in accurate detail because of the nature of the central nervous system. First, the separation and examination of a single nerve fiber is too delicate a procedure to be attempted in experiments on living humans. Second, in the central nervous system the myelinated nerve fibers are closely packed, so even if the procedure were not delicate and dangerous, it would nevertheless demand the greatest skill and patience.

Consequently, the primary sources of information are experiments on live animals, the dissection of bodies, both human and animal, and laboratory experiments with tissue. The information I have read and heard discussed by physicians interested in the disease suggests that MS isn't studied in live animals other than man because other animals are not susceptible to the disease. If true, this is a dubious distinction for man! Researchers are due a full measure of respect in addition to gratitude for they are essentially working on a problem which cannot be observed directly. Furthermore, the time of onset of the disease usually is known imprecisely, the activity of the disease can be charted only in gross terms, and the symptoms, when taken singly as they usually appear, typically tend to suggest something other than MS. So the necessarily indirect route to diagnosis of MS is a further frustration to the researchers, not to mention the practicing physician.

Earlier you may have noted some aggressive reaction to the information that indicated my wife and daughter were subjected to incalculable anguish by living with the knowledge that I had MS while I remained ignorant of the fact. When finally the doctor informed me and, nearly three years later, I told my wife, then the horror story began to unfold. The literature my family had been exposed to in attempts to cope with this secret was, as one of my neurologists put it: "horrible, misleading, and inaccurate even in the texts in medical school."

Previously it has been indicated that my exposure to books and articles on MS produced only a mild emotional reaction since most of the summaries of research were devoid of fear-inducing terms. But apparently even the literature from the Multiple Sclerosis Society in the early 1960's carried a heavy emphasis on the inevitability of the patient becoming a disabled, bedridden patient. My family waited through twelve terrifying years and symptom after symptom anticipating the inevitable trauma which would incapacitate. Now we find that the picture was inaccurate as a prognosis. Since having faced this same, not necessarily valid, prediction for the past three years, my insight into the torture endured by my family has deepened. I wish there were some way to return unwarped the years my wife and daughter spent unnecessarily burdened with a secret based on erroneous information.

One book on MS states that the clinical course of the disease is exceptionally variable and suggests five main types. One type is characterized by a swift succession of lesions accompanied by observable symptoms—an acute type of MS. This acute type results in a variety of conditions, ranging from a nearly complete recovery to death within a few weeks. The second type discussed is apparently the standard type. It is characterized by a series of attacks over a period of years and then the condition progresses to incapacitation. This second type is the standard basis for information about MS, or was so through the 1960's. The third variety of MS is similar to the second except that the attacks do not always appear to be MS attacks, and the diagnosis is difficult to make. The fourth type of MS suggested is characterized either by attacks of short duration or long intervals between the appearance of symptoms. This type is often referred to as "burning out" in time, leaving the patient with few traces of the symptoms. The final class of MS, according to this scheme, is symptomless, even though myelin is being destroyed in classic MS fashion.

One of my neurologists has a four-part scheme for describing conditions of MS. His is the analysis I prefer, and it is the one referred to later on in the book. He begins with type 1 in which the patient hardly knows there is anything wrong. Occasional attacks bring only slight symptoms, if any. Type 2 is more severe, yet the patient may remain ambulatory. This type is also characterized as appearing and receding like an iceberg bobbing up and down: old symptoms float into and out of consciousness, or recur, at unpredictable times and with a variety of degrees of intensity. New attacks occur from time to time. This type can end in a "burning out" or can progress to a type 3 or 4, although seldom to type 4. Type 3 is more severe than type 2, typically striking the legs and rendering the patient non-ambulatory but readily mobile via wheelchair. There is an indeterminate phase between types 2 and 3 during which the patient requires a cane for assistance in walking. Type 4 is the most severe and, apparently, is predictable within a few months of the initial diagnosis. This type of MS renders the patient essentially immobile.

Any of these current characterizations of MS is somewhat less frightening than the earlier idea that MS was unrelentingly progressive and inevitably disabling. This does not mean that MS can now be dismissed as a relatively minor and insignificant condition. But perhaps not every MS patient and family need be subjected to the earlier, gloomy picture.

Before moving on to deal with particular signs and symptoms of multiple sclerosis, it should be pointed out that geography would appear to play an important part in the incidence of MS. In general, the temperate zones harbor a higher likelihood of contracting the disease than does the equatorial zone. Your best bet for contracting MS seems to be living among advanced economic groups who endure cold winters. And, paradoxically, this disease haunts cleaner or more sanitary populaces. It is fitting that a paradox should arise so early in these considerations for several more lurk ahead.

Failure to mention some information about the nervous system would be a major omission, since portions of it are the scenes of attack by MS. The human nervous system can be characterized by means of dichotomies:

central vs. peripheral; sensory vs. motor; central vs. autonomic; and somatic vs. visceral. Perhaps a word about each of these dichotomies would be helpful in developing a concept of how the nervous system is affected by MS.

The central nervous system consists of the brain, brain stem and spinal column. The central nervous system controls the switching circuits, logic decisions and innumerable other mysterious processes which are called thinking. The peripheral nervous system, on the other hand, is more like a network of transmission lines. The peripheral system has two main functions: to transmit sensations to the central system and to transmit impulses or information from the central system to the skin, as well as to some areas deep inside the body. The nerves which lead into the central nervous system are called afferent fibers and are of a variety of kinds. The larger fibers have a myelin covering and transmit impulses rapidly. The smaller fibers are not myelinated, and transmit slower. Both the fast and the slow fibers carry impulses indicating heat, cold, and pain. Neurologists suggest that the peripheral nerves themselves are never involved in multiple sclerosis, which is a disease solely of the central nervous system.

Another dichotomy is composed of the motor neural system and the sensory neural system. Symptoms of a motor neural system attacked by multiple sclerosis can be varied. Again it is not the motor nerves themselves, but rather their extensions into the central system which are affected. Symptoms of a defective motor neural system include absence of abdominal reflexes, uncoordinated movements called ataxia, weakness in the limbs, leg jerkiness, spasticity, and some reflexes may become more pronounced. In contrast, the affected sensory system may offer the following symptoms: impaired kinesthetic perception, that is, not knowing where your hands, feet, knees, etc. are without looking; numbness, hypersensitivity, and coldness may occur in several places; the sensation of a limb falling asleep; and lost sensation of vibration.

A third dichotomy of the nervous system is autonomic vs. central. Having already mentioned symptoms indicating that the central nervous system is involved in multiple sclerosis, we now check on the autonomic system which includes both the sympathetic and the parasympathetic systems. Insult to the autonomic nerve system can create impotence, dizziness, and inability to control bladder function.

The fourth dichotomy assignable to the nervous system consists of the somatic and the visceral. The somatic nerves serve the trunk and limbs of the body. The visceral nerves serve the organs of the body. Clearly, as we have seen, the somatic nerves, or rather the central nerve carriers of the somatic nerve impulses, are involved in multiple sclerosis. Apparently those portions of the central system which transmit visceral nerve messages may also be invaded by multiple sclerosis, as you may discern in the chapters ahead.

With these subsystems of the nervous system laid out, perhaps the episodes in the chapters ahead will be somewhat more understandable. The main idea to keep in mind is the neurologists' firm assertion that it is the central nervous system which is involved in MS.

Perhaps you can imagine the broad range of symptoms, if not the myriad specific problems, which can be generated by a disease dancing about these dichotomies. If you cannot quite conjure up a problem for the patient, do not despair, some good examples await you. As one text on demyelination states, the demyelinating disorders often result in "bizarre clinical and pathologic manifestations."

The patient as well as his family, friends, and acquaintances are often astonished, perhaps dumbfounded by the sudden change in character of the patient's symptoms. When it is realized that many symptoms are invisible, some suspicion is aroused about the validity of the patient's complaints. Perhaps a realization of the cause of the symptoms will enable the reader to accept them more readily.

3
About Physicians and Families

Having endured the strange manifestations of multiple sclerosis for more than a decade before being informed of the diagnosis, I have some reflections which may sound like advice to physicians. If nothing more, perhaps these reflections will impress upon those physicians who tend to believe otherwise that multiple sclerosis is manifest in both physical and psychological symptoms. Not only is the central nervous system involved, but thoughts about that system are inevitable. With such complete involvement of the patient in the consequences of the disease, emotional factors loom as large as do physical factors.

But it would be unfair to offer advice without apologies to my own physician who, after all, did successfully guide the diagnostic process to an accurate conclusion. Many acquaintances who suffer MS state that their physicians apparently didn't know what the problem was. Even worse, one fellow, a recent acquaintance, visited several neurologists who seemed unable to make the diagnosis; at least they did not do so. Another man, it is reported, appeared at an MS center and announced to the physician, "I have multiple sclerosis." Asked whether he had been diagnosed, he said, "No. But I have been making the rounds of so many physicians and neurologists that I have made the diagnosis myself." His diagnosis was accurate.

So if any advice offered here seems harsh, it is nevertheless meant to be couched in admiration for the physician who can make the diagnosis. However, for neurologists who ought to be able to diagnose MS, and who ought to turn in their specialty license if they cannot, perhaps my friend's term "yo-yo" is an apt expression.

No doubt one wonders how any patient could be so naive as to enable a physician to hide the diagnosis of a condition like MS from him for over a decade. But as I have indicated, the nature of the condition often leads to a series of apparently discrete, independent medical problems. If physicians, even neurological specialists, can fail to identify the condition which connects such problems as symptoms of a disease, perhaps it is not difficult to imagine how a patient could be diverted from the truth for a long time. You just face each problem as it arises and become distressed over having so many different problems.

It is, however, conscious keeping of the diagnosis from the patient by the physician which is an issue for me. I base my opposition to this deception on five grounds: first, the patient has a right to take action about his body in the full light of information known by his physician; second, there are actions of a legal nature, such as the drawing of wills and disposition of estates which are made more urgent by the diagnosis; third, the patient has a right to try to cope with the real physical situation rather than being hounded by the possibility that his symptoms are psychosomatic; fourth, the patient should be able to inform other physicians of his condition in case of an emergency; and fifth, the patient should have the responsibility for deciding whether or not to burden his loved ones with a diagnosis such as multiple sclerosis, rather than, as in my case, having only the family privy to the diagnosis.

In the first instance, the patient's right to take action about his body in the full light of information known by the physician, alternative courses of action are closed to the MS patient who is not told the diagnosis. For example, his search for what would perhaps be better medical opinion is circumscribed by lack of knowledge to direct his search. Based on the only information available, that gained from observation of my own symptoms, I could have sought outside advice from a specialist in numbness, or a practitioner in false heart attacks, but none was known to me.

The idea of a search for additional or better medical advice brings to mind a vivid memory of a situation which occurred a generation ago. I was a graduate student and a research assistant at The University of Chicago at the time. One day the professor for whom I worked walked into the statistics laboratory, my place of work. He sat down and said to me, "My son is dying; he has cancer." The professor then wept, and I sat dumbfounded, unable to think of any response. After he and his son had been informed of the diagnosis, he had had several specialists flown in to confirm the diagnosis. This was not a reflection on the competency of the physician who made the original diagnosis. Rather, it was a father's attempt to leave no stone unturned in a search for hope. No physician has the right to block such a search by refusing information or advising against disclosure to the patient.

Another example of options closed to an uninformed patient is the opportunity to participate in research on the condition, either during his lifetime or following it. Donating one's body to research on a particular disease is extremely difficult when the name of that disease is unknown to the donor. And volunteering for experiments during one's lifetime is similarly hindered when the disabling condition is unknown to you. Within two years of the disclosure to me I was involved as a volunteer subject in a study of people with multiple sclerosis.

The second ground from which to contend that the patient has a right to know of the diagnosis of multiple sclerosis is that there are legal actions which the patient may want to initiate. Wills, for example, require some witnessed assertion of competence. This kind of competence, as various episodes related later suggest, may sometimes be subject to varying degrees of doubt. Regardless of the question of competence is the possible urgency to have legal documents drawn.

The third instance involves the patient's right to cope with the real situation rather than being in an increasingly unsettling state, believing that his problems are psychosomatic. Here different potential actions are thwarted. Occasionally, when faced by a colleague or friend who believes he is a psychiatrist, and who reacts to one of your obvious symptoms by suggesting it is psychosomatic, it becomes increasingly difficult to avoid wondering whether he is right. Even when your physical-problem-oriented physician condescends to assure you that "this is not hysterical," the mental relief is only temporary.

Short of the psychosomatic problem lies the patient's right to exercise his full capacity in dealing with the symptomatic physical conditions. There seems to be no long-term value in dissipating energy in fruitless worry and despair when the insulting condition calls for energy to be husbanded; there is full measure of concern over just the physical problems. Furthermore, a frank disclosure of the diagnosis might free the physician sufficiently to enable him to prescribe, occasionally, a drug which could relieve symptoms such as the rest-disturbing leg jerks at night. Also involved in the exercise of full powers is the possibility that the unconscious works to develop alternative neural pathways for messages and substitute patterns for thought in the brain. These very real possibilities would seem to be dependent on initial conscious knowledge of the offending neurological condition.

The fourth ground for complaint about the physician withholding the diagnosis from the patient involves emergency situations, particularly those occurring when the patient is out of town. As you will see, we became involved in such an emergency. At the time I was unable to shed light on the problem because of my lack of information about the basic diagnosis.

The fifth situation, informing the family of the diagnosis without informing the patient, is the most distressing of all. It can generate unbridled anger in the patient when he learns of it. When finally it seemed time to me to inform my wife of the diagnosis, about two years after my having learned of it, her response was unbelievable. She said she and our daughter had known for about a dozen years. I was surprised. "Amazed" is perhaps a more accurate characterization. I was also remorseful that they had had to undergo the stress and strain of not only the grim prospects of our lifestyle but also the containment of that secret.

However, my remorse was short-lived in the initial confessional situation, for much of my wife's pent-up emotion, frustration, and anger was vented on me immediately. As the torrent of abuse flowed over my prostrate form, I asked myself what was happening. As Kay heard later, "Here I was a 'sick and dying man,' and for no reason at all you were giving me hell." It was a scene of classic farce, except that I quickly realized what must have been happening. Then the extent of my family's suffering struck me like a gigantic, overwhelming and suffocating pillow.

Two or three years later we came across some of our daughter's high school report cards. Those from the year she and her mother learned of my condition were of particular interest. They contained comments from two teachers, each of whom reported that she at times acted quite out of character, seeming preoccupied and not the capable, likeable student they thought they knew so well. No wonder! A youngster might easily become preoccupied while sharing with her mother the secret that her father was suffering from a dreadful, progressive, incapacitating disease, as the literature of that time presented MS to be.

At the moment of my discovery that they knew what had been withheld from me, it was clear the torment which must have visited my family relentlessly over the years; torment which I probably would have attempted to spare them given the opportunity; agony which could at least have been postponed, perhaps softened by better information from a more fully informed source; despair which could possibly have been shared rather than being endured in loneliness, and at an unknown emotional price. I have since learned that at one point my wife said to the physician: "You had damned well better be right about this diagnosis or I will sue you." She must have been furiously frustrated.

Although the language is stronger than some I have used, a friend of mine has represented the opinion of many by saying, "Who do physicians think they are, God? Making decisions like that without consulting the patient! It is outrageous." Later events confirmed my initial reaction upon learning that my family had been apprised of my condition years earlier: I would not have wished such a burden upon them, and would have gone to some lengths to have spared them the dreadful ordeal through which they lived.

One must realize that the dozen years between the initial diagnosis and the announcement of that diagnosis to the patient were years during which more definite information about MS was garnered via research. Thus it could be argued that the patient would have had no alternatives to explore, that the best information available at that time was brought to bear. Similarly, no doubt it could be contended that no aids to coping were available. And clearly, it has been argued, that one option open to the physician is to shield the patient from the trauma of knowing about a disease presumed to be progressive, and probably inevitably incapacitating.

The first of these arguments is the easiest for me to entertain, but it is neither certain nor clear to me that more or better information would not have been available. Furthermore, even in recent years, after he had revealed the diagnosis, the physician failed to initiate procedures which had come into practice. The second argument, about coping, I reject out of hand. Anyone with a will to live can deal more effectively with a dreaded disease when informed about it than when he must grope in ignorance, at the same time struggling against the psychological trauma of considering that his problems may be psychosomatic.

Continuing for a moment my response to the second argument, let me recite a coping situation which I observed from the vantage point of a participant. Among our friends was a widower with a teen-aged daughter. One summer, while she was studying in Europe for six weeks with one of her high school classes, he was stricken with three types of cancer. Moved into a cancer research hospital, his condition was brought under control through combinations of drugs and blood transfusions. We marveled at the skill of the physicians in manipulating drug dosages to control the immediate effects of the condition.

After some weeks our friend asked to be moved from the hospital. At that time he was once again a lively conversationalist with a large number of daily visitors, so he was enjoying life to some extent. He was moved to the nearby home of a friendly family and ensconced in a second floor bedroom. I participated in the move and in one or more of the semiweekly trips to the hospital for blood transfusions.

So far as we could tell he should have died before the drug regime was established. But there he was, living away from the hospital, in good spirits, and with enough strength to feed and dress himself. With assistance he was even able to negotiate the stairs, although slowly. One of our mutual friends inquired about the patient one day. When I had told the tale, the friend said, "What's going on? What keeps him going?" My reply was: "I don't really know, but his daughter is due to return in four or five days." "Ooooooh," replied my friend, "Look out," and I knew what he meant.

The patient lived to see his daughter return, then died within a few days. Such stories are legion and support the contention that one can cope with disease to unbelievable limits—but not unless you know what it is you are battling. At least, in all the cases known to me, the successful battle was waged by a person who knew the nature of his condition.

The third argument, that the physician is protecting the patient by shielding him from the awful truth, is no argument at all when one considers the burden imposed upon those who are not ill, the family. Indeed! Who is entitled to give the diagnosis to the family but not to the patient? Who has the right to make such decisions affecting the lives of both the patient and his family without consulting the patient? Furthermore, whatever problems burden the family in such a situation, the patient has a severe problem at times in knowing who he is, in continuing an identity which can accommodate a succession of medical problems which make little sense and which are identified but remain essentially unexplained by the physician.

In closing these introductory remarks about the responsibilities and rights of physicians, patients, and families, one additional incident which occurred very recently seems relevant. It is my fortune to have blood of type "O" and with a "negative" Rh factor. This, it was said many years ago, is known as "universal donor" blood. True or not, for twenty years my blood was sought. Those years, it seems to me, embrace a period of time prior to the current, highly organized blood drives by blood banks, and extend into the period of my illness. In any case, since learning of my condition I have checked with a local blood bank, inquiring whether it would accept my blood. When the attendant learned that I suffered from multiple sclerosis, he quickly closed the conversation after saying they could not accept my blood because of my condition. This leads me to wonder what problems or injury might have been caused by the use of my blood during earlier years when I was afflicted but unaware that the malady was multiple sclerosis.

Perhaps I feel better now, having aired some of the frustration felt over a decade-and-a-half; at least some psychiatrists and clinical psychologists would think that I might. However, no difference in feeling seems detectable, but perhaps relief is there anyway.

Perhaps these pages are a rationalization. It is hoped, however, that more has been accomplished. If others are no more knowledgeable than I was about multiple sclerosis, perhaps they will learn something about the disease in the pages ahead. Certainly the public is being made aware of it through endeavors such as the "Athletes vs. Multiple Sclerosis" campaign. But awareness is different from knowledge, and both are intended outcomes for those who read through this material. Chapter 2 has plunged us into information about the disease. We now turn to an exploration of a variety of conditions which emanate from the basic difficulty. These are discussed in the chapters which follow.

4
Early Signs and Recalled Oddities

The traceable chain of events which revealed my affliction with multiple sclerosis began in an operating room where, under local anesthesia, a sebaceous cyst was being removed from the back side of my upper right arm. I was 36 years old. It was March 1959. The date in the record is March 27 but it is not clear whether this was the date of the operation or of the removal of stitches.

My physician, who was also a reasonably good surgeon, was allowing a resident to perform the procedure. When I mentioned that the incision could be felt, they administered more anesthetic, Novocain as I recall. This was repeated when I suggested that some feeling was still noticeable. The surgeon remarked that it was unlikely that further pain would be felt, indicating that no feeling should have been noted after the initial injection.

My return visit to the office for the removal of a stitch or two was remarkable because of two things I said. First: "The outside edge of my right hand and little finger is numb." Second: "I think your assistant may have severed a nerve." This volley brought instant response. First we established the exact location of the numbness. Next we checked the strength of my right hand grip. The physician assured me that no nerve had been severed, and he continued to check this condition for months until other, more severe symptoms appeared.

My thoughts drifted idly to the possibility that the chemical anesthetic had insulted the nerve. With nothing better to go on, this vague belief persisted until finally I was informed of the MS diagnosis more than a decade later. In fact, before revealing the diagnosis to me the physician asked what I thought was wrong, and I recited this belief about the anesthetic. The numbness persists to this day, intruding into my consciousness from time to time, depending on both the state of the condition and the state of my consciousness. This was the first in a series of events that resembled each other much as one link in a chain resembles another: all appeared suddenly, seemed inexplicable, faded from consciousness, and floated in and out of consciousness on an apparently random schedule.

The symptom most closely paralleling the first appeared late one afternoon in a hotel room near the Western Reserve University campus (now Case-Western Reserve), in Cleveland. The time was December 1961, and the event precipitated the myelogram done in January 1962. For about seven years I was privileged to be a consultant to W.R.U.'s Division of Research in Medical Education, a position which accorded the opportunity to work with many of the remarkable faculty members of that school of medicine. It also required long, often tough-minded sessions, morning, afternoon and night, with occasional luncheon and dinner sessions wedged in. On this particular day we had finished an afternoon work session and I had returned to my room for a brief rest and shower before undertaking cocktails, dinner, and an evening session.

As I lay resting on the bed, a sensation of numbness suddenly became apparent in the top of the thigh of my right leg. It moved, or extended perceptibly downward toward the knee in a thin line. Thinking it might be a bug of some kind, I checked the skin area but found nothing. Completely puzzled by this sensation, I lay quietly concentrating on it and wondering what could be happening. Needless to say, the search, through my ignorance about such matters, resolved nothing. Time whirled forward impishly and, since there seemed to be no physical impairment, I arose to undertake and complete the schedule for the day. No doubt my effectiveness was less than maximum the remainder of that trip, for the strange sensation persisted. It was worrisome.

Upon returning to Chicago I scheduled an appointment with my physician to report this numbness. Thence began one of the more irksome diagnostic routines used in this condition. The object is to determine whether or not there is a change in sensibility from one area to another on the skin. Two, sometimes three, instruments are used: a needle-like object with which you are stabbed gently, meaning that the skin is not broken but not meaning that the process is free from pain; a feather, or similar object formed hurriedly from absorbent tissue paper, is used to tickle skin areas in an effort to elicit some of the hundreds of reflexes with which the human body is endowed. The third instrument is pointed like the needle, but weighted; it seemed sometimes to be on the handle end of the hammer used to test knee reflexes. Whatever it was, it was used in a sort of combined function; testing reflexes like the feather, as it was dragged across the abdomen for example, but hurting as the skin was scratched by the sometimes unnecessarily sharp point, thus enabling the patient to report that he could or could not feel pain.

The needle routine goes as follows: "Can you feel this

(jab)?" "Yes;" or, "Does this (jab) feel sharp or dull?"
"Sharp;" or, "Does this (jab) feel different from this
(jab)?" "No. They are both sharp." This procedure, done
at high speed, enabled my physician to trace a path of
dulled sensation, perhaps numbness, from a point about
belt high on my spine downward and to the right across the
top of the right buttock, continuing down the hip, across
the top of the thigh, where I had first felt the sensation,
ending in a right-hand swirl from the inside of the knee
area, toward and perhaps under the kneecap. This procedure was repeated many times in the ensuing months.
Once or twice the physician drew the path on my skin using
some kind of soft marker. This *objet d'art* was then displayed to another physician who apparently validated the
belief that a page from a neuro-anatomy book had just been
reproduced on a live subject. (Throughout, words like "apparently" and phrases such as "it seemed as though" are
used in connection with the various physicians' activities
for the simple reason that none of them ever told me anything substantial.)

Whether this symptom ever disappeared or reappeared
is a moot question. When you test for numbness in a
portion of your leg by rubbing with a hand which has a
streak of numbness itself, it is difficult to decide much
about the leg. It does seem that cold weather alerts me to
the probability that the original numbness persists.

But symptoms of the Cleveland episode included more
than a portion of one leg. As may have been suggested by
the preceding discussion, the symptoms extended to the loss
of reflexes in the abdominal region. Lying on the examining
table watching a feather being dragged across the abdomen,
it was clear that there was no reflex action visible. Of
course this set of reflexes as well as the sharp-dull contrast
was always tested with my eyes closed prior to my observation of the repeated feather test.

Two things are worth noting in retrospect. First, some symptoms were localizing in the abdominal and lower trunk area. As you will find later, this trend was indeed developing, and can, perhaps, be understood in the light of the nature of multiple sclerosis. Second, and perhaps more relevant to the physician's handling of my case, the abdominal reflexes were the first symptom which can be truly said to have returned to normal, so far as I know. The submerging-emerging characteristic of MS in what we called type 2 in the earlier chapter, seems to have been unknown to my physician. When the abdominal reflexes returned, and other physical symptoms seemed to have disappeared in 1973, I was scheduled for a reassessment by a prominent neurologist. Incidentally, he had been a resident in neurology in the same institution when the then chief of neurology had confirmed my diagnosis twelve or thirteen years earlier. Not a specialist in MS, he wrote to my physician that there was no reason to change the diagnosis although he believed the patient was not as severely affected as he, the patient, seemed to believe. My complaints stemmed from symptoms which are to be discussed later and from the recurring nature of other symptoms. The neurologist's report seemed to stem from ignorance of or dismissal of the waxing and waning characteristic of type 2 MS and from the belief that short of types 3 or 4, most symptoms of MS were insignificant. Let me assure you that they are not!

So much, then, for early symptoms which are rather easily consolidated in the recorded history of my bout with MS. What, then, can be said in support of the contention that the victim of MS is ticketed for this eventuality by very early teen age? Did I escape all symptoms until near the age of forty? I think not.

A pair of events from late 1945 and New Year's Day of 1946 have always been vivid in my memory. In 1974, the speaker at the annual luncheon of the Chicago Chapter of the National Multiple Sclerosis Society mentioned the possibility that a virus might be involved in the disease. Until that day I had never associated the two early events in anything but a chronological stream. But now they take on the semblance of a cause-effect relationship. There is little to report about either event, so I will be brief.

Late in 1945, probably in December, our unit, and very likely all service personnel on Guam at the time, were ordered to receive an influenza shot. Whether this was a precaution for troops being returned to the States before the end of winter, or an experiment to test the effectiveness of a vaccine, I do not know. At the time it was rumored that this was an experiment. In any event, I recall making my way back to my bed, a distance not exceeding one hundred yards, flopping down, and awakening about noon the following day after approximately twenty-four hours of minimally interrupted sack time. The only thing that ever approximated that in my life was a bout with ptomaine poisoning, but then I arose periodically to vomit and take an antidote. So this episode is reasonably clear in my memory, having been the subject of ever-so-many "when I was in the service" recollections over the years. Since that time, and continuing to this day, I have suffered what surely was a consequence of the shot. Cold sores have plagued me ever since, even appearing occasionally in summer. And they are large, nasty affairs.

The second episode, which I connected to the first only recently after learning something about MS, occurred on New Year's Day, 1946, just a few weeks after the flu shot episode. We had been assigned temporary duty on neighboring Saipan, or Tinian, I forget which, and found ourselves without specific jobs on the beautiful, warm, sunny morning of New Year's Day, 1946. Nearby we found a tennis court and someone located four racquets and some tennis balls. Although I considered myself proficient at the game, to my dismay I found myself often swinging and missing the ball completely. Some attempts found me striking the ball with the wooden frame of the racquet, but what was most puzzling, distressing and aggravating was my obvious inability to hit the ball regularly with the tennis racquet. There was, of course, some banter about the day after the night before, and barbs about "I thought you said you were on the high school tennis team," etc. I found the episode basically distressing and puzzling. My current suspicion is that I was having or had had an MS attack. Further, this probability is now associated firmly in my mind with the possibility that the attack may have been precipitated by the flu shot a few short weeks earlier.

One further example of an oddity which may well have been an early sign that MS had invaded my body involved feelings about my legs. Of course the legs have been considered a major focal point for "real" MS, and are the symbol of type 3 MS. More is said about the affliction of my legs later but here I should like to recount a recurring episode from years before the diagnosis was made, and perhaps two decades or more before the diagnosis was revealed to me.

Throughout my life I have been an ardent walker. Perhaps it was a habit ingrained by accompanying my father, upon occasion, on his walk from our home to our farm and return, a total distance of about 15 miles. Perhaps it was a natural consequence of the fact that I always seemed to be marching in a band for some celebration, event, or contest. Having earned a position in the high school band upon entering grade 7, six years were spent marching in contests in Des Moines, Cleveland, Holland (Michigan), Detroit, etc., in addition to parades on Memorial Day, Armistice Day, July Fourth, etc. Then I graduated to the University of Michigan Band which practiced marching five days a week during football season, and we not only marched at the games, but paraded to and from the stadium on Saturday afternoons.

These activities plus bicycle riding and a lively interest in a variety of sports, unaccompanied by any remarkable skill, made leg power a significant part of my life. Perhaps it is understandable that, when an odd feeling invaded one or both legs at unspecified times, a sort of dullness of sensation as I recall, the thought occurred to me that my legs must be wearing out. Although the times of these occurrences are apparently gone from memory, recollection of the kinds of thoughts engendered seem relatively available for reconstruction. The idea that my legs were wearing out was never pursued, since the specter appeared of a peg leg being worn down, or something like that, and it was obvious that my feet and legs could not literally be worn down in that sense. This impasse always brought my conscious thought about the matter to an end, leaving me with only idle curiosity about the strange feeling.

In more recent years, though prior to learning of the diagnosis, my response to such episodes was similar to that of earlier times: walk and exercise the legs. But the more recent response was made in the light of a vague, semiconscious belief that the legs could be stirred from a partial sleep into which they were falling. Much earlier there was not a concentrated concern, but rather a passing curiosity which was aroused only by the recurrence of the odd feeling.

In summary then, upon reflection it seems highly probable that attacks of multiple sclerosis have been a part of my life since shortly after age twenty, and possibly longer. As my wife once said in a tender moment, "You may never have known a normal day. That's too bad."

If the foregoing were classified as physical signs, there remain signs which could be called non-physical. Let me share the history of a few.

During the 1960's, but subsequent to the physician's secret diagnosis of my MS, two changes occurred which seem worth noting. The first, briefly stated, is that I became very introspective, at least in my private hours. The second, more readily verifiable, requires a bit of background.

At some point during my introspective period it occurred to me that many men probably never manage to attain a level of emotional maturity much beyond that of a healthy 15-year-old. I would not argue the point, but this contention has been sustained by confirming incidents related by others to whom I have suggested it. In my own case, without conjecture about the ages involved, my wife and I agreed at one time that my emotional age had changed. She said she thought that I had regressed in the early sixties. After considerable thought it seemed clear that she was right; a substantial shift in my emotional age had occurred. We also agree that considerable forward progress has been made by me since that hazily specified time.

That emotional regression occurred there can be little doubt. That it happened during the period when several attacks of MS occurred is also nearly indisputable. Whether there is a causal connection I cannot tell. One thing is clear: a causal connection did not cross my mind until reading the papers from a symposium, "Clinical Psychological Services to Multiple Sclerosis Patients," presented at the 1974 meeting of the American Psychological Association in New Orleans. A summary of research on emotional and personality correlates of MS in the paper by Susan Andrews of the University of Wisconsin Center-Waukesha County and Sacred Heart Rehabilitation Hospital suggested a possible causal connection between emotional factors and MS. The investigators have been seeking causes for the onset of MS while my private case study would have the MS causal of emotional regression. Needless to say, I shall not attempt to dispute the research accomplished;

rather I simply report a conclusion from some quaint musings.

Additional possible evidence that regression takes place in MS is offered from our own experience. One evident characteristic of many severely handicapped adults Kay and I have observed is selfishness. This takes the form of greed at the table where many show no consideration for others, in fact they sometimes are oblivious to the presence of others. When viewed as behavior by adults this is almost inexcusable. When considered as possible regression to a state of development marked by parallel, independent activity, a state in which interactive activity is not conceivable, the greedy behavior is more understandable, even acceptable.

Somewhat more recently, perhaps in 1970, a rather strange thing happened to me; I found myself saying things about myself that were true, yet new to me. The occasion was an informal meeting between students and the faculty of a specialized program within the department. There were probably ten to a dozen students and three or four faculty members present.

Ostensibly the purpose of the meeting was to acquaint the students more fully with the faculty. The students desired to hear briefly about any research we were then doing, to learn something of our personal habits, beliefs, interests, etc., and in general to get to know us better. By the time my turn came to say a few words, a pattern of presentation had evolved. Following that pattern, I told a little of my educational background and turned to some of my personal characteristics before moving on to tell about current research interests.

I found myself saying that I had a very short attention span. Consequently the students would find me with three or four activities in various states of completion at any given time. In this fashion my short attention span was, so to speak, accommodated. Whether or not this portion of my presentation was of any interest to the students, it interested me a great deal. In the days that followed I returned to consider the fact of my short span of attention.

In speaking of my short span of attention, I am speaking in relative terms. My attention span did not approximate the briefness of a few seconds which is the span of some youngsters when first entering public school. But the effects stemming from a relatively short span are just as telling. For example, in the early 1960's when able to relax and concentrate on the task, my reading speed was slightly in excess of 4,000 words a minute with excellent comprehension. This is not an unusual accomplishment among my colleagues, who may read critically several books and manuscripts each week. At the time under discussion, that is, following the informal meeting with students, my reading rate was between 200 and 300 words per minute. Using 4,000 as 100 per cent, my reading speed of 300 words per minute was a drop to about 8 per cent. In these terms over 90 per cent of my reading efficiency had been lost. Most of the loss seems attributable to an inability to focus attention on the task at hand.

In this same vein it is interesting, though disheartening, to recall the task on which my attention was focused the day that double-vision struck. The problem requiring my attention was a complicated one. It was an attempt to program for a small computer a sophisticated statistical procedure used in analyzing some kinds of research data. Not only was the set of computations complicated, but the computer was too small to handle all the data and do all the computations. Consequently, the program was being arranged so the computer would accept the original data, do some computations and punch cards. These cards were then fed back in with another section of the computations. Eventually the program was completed in three sections.

The task of completing this computer program required many days. Each morning it was necessary for me to sit down, recall the point already reached in the program, load into my memory exactly what would be happening to each set of numbers inside the computer and then move ahead with the new programming. Sometimes it would require nearly an hour of concentrated thought first thing in the morning before the first new instruction for the computer program could be written.

There seems to be no handy way to express the per cent loss of that kind of concentration. I can only say that the loss was enormous. When part of your ego support as well as advancement in your profession is heavily dependent on the levels of skill and concentration suggested above, the loss of a significant degree of such concentration can be devastating. Fortunately I cannot report negative consequences which are severe enough to be labeled "devastating," but they were indeed severe.

Another incident, involving an extensively burned young man, may further suggest what lack of concentration can mean. Having learned that this man liked to play chess, I invited him to tell me when he felt like having a game. This he did a week or so later, and so we began. After five or six moves he sat alternately motionless and shaking his head. Finally he said: "Let's quit now. I just don't have any ideas." He realized his inability at that time to generate an attacking pattern for the game. I shall always believe that his temporary inability to "have any ideas" stemmed from the constant and enormous distraction of his attention from the game to his healing wounds. To have an idea is not a simple task, and distractions from intense concentration can thwart the process.

Adjustment is a key process in learning to live with MS. Perhaps my most agonizing adjustment came in my professional life. Two estimates of my loss of potential have already been mentioned, the dramatic drops in reading speed and focus of attention. Saying that the adjustment was rather severe but not professionally devastating leads me to suggest an impressionistic characterization of my plight. Further advancement was denied, and even salary increments arrived but occasionally and in dribbles. I came to be treated as a sort of village idiot: suffered, acknowledged, used for menial tasks only, and entrusted with little or nothing. The only consolation was that I operated in a high-class village.

There is yet to be discussed the episode which may have been the high point of my early experiences with MS. The episode revolves around the myelogram. According to my very old and very large Webster's, *myelo* is a combining form meaning *the marrow* or the *spinal cord*, a derivative of the Greek *myelos* meaning marrow. *Gram* is also a combination form used to form nouns meaning *something written* or *drawn*, also from Greek. When combined, these two combining forms compose the noun *myelogram*, something to be avoided if at all possible. Myelogram really stands for an x-ray picture, or series of x-ray pictures of the spine. It also seems to stand for the procedure followed in order to obtain the pictures.

Such pictures can be very important both for locating the cause of a suspected condition and for eliminating a condition as a basis for diagnosis. In my case the physician ordered it following the Cleveland episode. Numbness, or altered sensation as I learned to say, had struck the outer edge of my right hand and small finger, as well as a nerve leading from the small of my back down and around the leg to the kneecap area. It is with reasonable confidence that, in retrospect, I say the physician had these and other symtoms in mind when he ordered the myelogram.

Fortunately, perhaps, a friend with sereve back trouble had unwittingly alerted me to the dangers of a myelogram. Before my symptoms suggested a myelogram, Con had had one as part of the diagnostic process to determine a cause of his back problem. At that time he said "Watch out for the headache afterwards." Further conversation led me to believe that the aftermath of a myelogram was a severe, pounding headache which defied all but the most powerful pain killers.

Con's warning proved to be unnecessary in my case some years later. After the procedure and my return to bed, I lay motionless, monitoring areas of the brain where severe headaches had occurred in the past. This is not to suggest that I had been susceptible to severe headaches, only that the sites of the occasional ones were well remembered.

No pain could be detected. Throughout the day and evening I waited. No pain appeared. I would have been happier, however, had the physician not said that the procedure would be repeated after an interval of one day. You see, they withdraw some of your spinal fluid and replace it with a colored fluid which provides contrast for the x-ray pictures. My physician said: "They didn't put quite enough colored fluid in, so they have to do it over again." I have never quite believed that explanation, but what is a patient to do? All that aside, no headache appeared following the second myelogram, and I was greatly relieved.

But you should know about myelograms. As stated before, some of the spinal fluid is withdrawn and replaced by a colored fluid for x-ray purposes. The entire spinal column is x-rayed by segments. But there is only a small amount of colored fluid in the column, enough to fill a small section. Then how do the technicians x-ray the entire column? That's where the fun and games come.

You are placed face down, spread-eagle on a large table. I had the impression it was a large round table, but it probably was a standard rectangular x-ray table. The physician directing operations was reputed to be one of the best. She sounded very authoritative in the darkened room, and I was cowed, if not frightened. There must have been two additional persons in the room, one operating the table, the other the x-ray machine. It is difficult to know these things when only one voice is heard in the dark.

My physician informed me, I forget whether before or after the myelograms, that he was looking for a bone chip or anything else that might account for the episodes of numbness, or altered sensation. With this purpose, and the necessity for relying on a small amount of colored fluid to help in the x-ray photographing of sections of the spine, the procedure could have been deduced. For whatever reason, I did not foresee the procedure, and thus was dumbfounded and nearly paralyzed with apprehension when the table was tilted one way and another with me spread-eagled and not secured to it.

The crew was busy making the colored fluid move down the spine to the next location which was to be photographed. Obviously the table had to be tilted so that my head was down. Then, of course, it had to be tilted to one side or the other in order to place the fluid in just the right spot. I literally hung on by my fingers at times.

In addition to the tenseness from worrying about falling off the table, the physician in charge constantly reminded me: "Don't move! Lie perfectly still!" And these were issued as orders, delivered in a very loud, rather low and heavy female voice. She also directed one or two other persons who, as has been said, ran the table switches and took the x-rays. In the midst of this peculiar event in the darkness I had visions of the director floating about on one of those Hollywood director's chairs which seem to move effortlessly in all directions on the end of an hydraulic boom. Her voice came from first one direction then another, sometimes high above me. It was an experience not easily forgotten.

By the way, after the picture taking was finished the crew had to maneuver the fluid back to the top of the spine and then withdraw it. Perhaps you can imagine my feelings when told that the myelogram was to be repeated! But the headache never developed.

My physician informed me that no chip or other substance was found which might have caused the numbness. He never mentioned the cerebrospinal fluid which had been withdrawn, and I gave it no thought until recently. It is now my impression that particles of protein from demyelination of the brain have been found as trash in the spinal fluid of patients with MS. Recall also that antibodies which act on the central nervous system have been found in spinal fluid. This has caused me to wonder whether or not an examination was made of my spinal fluid after the myelogram. I suspect that it was, and that the evidence was useful in making the final diagnosis.

So much, then, for some of the early signs of MS as they appear to me in retrospect. The fact that nearly all of the strange events are seen only in this fragmented way is because I possessed no unifying concept for them until about three years ago. If any of these probable symptoms would recur, or if new symptoms were to appear, God forbid, they now would be assimilated readily into the concept MS. Previously they were seen only as isolated incidents, each of which was sufficiently interesting, peculiar, or traumatic to linger in memory with some freshness.

There was quite a different set of events which occurred relatively early in my bout with MS. Though some may say that these events had no connection with MS, I remain unable to agree with them. You may decide for yourself.

From time to time a person is led to realize the extent to which he is a creature as well as a human. Squirrels, who seem constantly to be hoarding food, are no match for some people engaged in the same endeavor; territorial rights are as real and fundamental to humans as to seals and dogs and tigers. In fact, I once observed that man's ability to conceptualize and transfer learning had led him to extend territorial rights to the time dimension of life; at least it seems so when trying to arrange a program involving two or more persons or when school faculties discuss amounts of time to be devoted to each subject.

But creatureness has a desirable and beneficial dimension, or so folklore has it. Have you never heard that persons, particularly youngsters, will develop a craving for food which contains a nutrient their diet has been lacking? My experience over a period of many years suggests that exercise too is sought when it is felt necessary, although the reason for the necessity may be no more a part of consciousness and rationality than is the craving for foods.

Most MS patients whom I met in a discussion group said they exercised. These people did so consciously and, typically, upon advice of a neurologist. All indicated that they exercised in order to preserve whatever strength and muscle tone they had, and in the hope that they might grow stronger in their afflicted limbs. Perhaps the most extreme case was that of a woman who exercised her legs while wearing five-pound weights around her ankles.

Since learning the nature of my affliction I too have exercised to maintain muscle tone and to increase strength in certain muscles. Some exercises designed to tighten the abdominal muscles also have been included. Creatureness, however, was manifest in the form of exercise many years before it would have been possible for me to know what I was doing in terms of MS. To have asked me why I was undertaking exercise would have been as fruitful as asking a dog why he trods in a circle in his bed before lying down.

The particular exercises undertaken were the first dozen or so from a book about yoga. I got as far as the headstand. Although the headstand never yielded to my efforts, I did spend a lot of time increasing the circulation to my head. The folded, locked-leg position was achieved to the point that it was almost comfortable. One of my favorites was standing on one leg while bending the other until parallel to the floor, holding the foot of the bent leg in the opposite hand while bending forward (or any other way you could) in an effort to touch the floor with the free hand. One has ample opportunity to learn to balance while trying to accomplish this exercise, especially when you alternate the legs on which you stand. Falling is unavoidable for a time.

One of the major forms of exercise which I attempted was learning to sail. Rowing a dinghy to and from the mooring, rigging the boat, and climbing forward to ride the bow while avoiding entanglement with the jib, provides oodles of exercise for arms and legs. Also involved is lots of practice at balancing. Handling the tiller and the mainsheet while maneuvering the boat provides additional exercise to numerous parts of the body.

Not entirely in preparation for sailing, but so in part, was my two-year escapade at the gymnasium. Several days each week an hour or so was spent jogging, working out on a contraption rigged to accommodate nine or ten types of weightlifting, exercising against the gravitational pull of my body mass, and swimming. It seems clear that fatigue, as a normal state, was in remission during this period. If it were not, I would scarcely have negotiated the climb from the basement locker room to the second-floor track.

My point here is that perhaps through some "instinct," in almost animal fashion, I began a series of exercises of which some would surely have been recommended had such recommendation not opened the door for inadvertent disclosure of my health problem. I often reflect on how uncanny was this phase of my life with MS.

So much for some of the early signs as seen in retrospect. That these events transpired, let there be no doubt. Whether it is appropriate to interpret them as part of the MS scheme may be debatable. So far as I am concerned, these events are less odd in the context of MS than in any other single explanation. In fact, no other one context capable of encompassing all these oddities has occured to me.

5
Weird Wonderments

There are myriad symptoms of multiple sclerosis. It is often said that each patient has a unique pattern of ailments and complaints. Whether or not this is possible or true is beyond the scope of consideration here. Certainly there are many common symptoms, and some of these are suggested in the next chapter. But among the problems I have encountered, several seem worthy of special consideration. These are here called "weird wonderments."

Such "special" attacks of MS demonstrate several points. First, they range widely over the functions they affect, again underscoring how a patient might easily believe that each new attack is an isolated, discrete phenomenon. Second, some of the malfunctions in an organ, limb, or system which result from an MS attack are apparently contradictory but such contradictory afflictions do arise in some situations stemming from MS. Third, the extent and recurrence of symptoms in type 2 MS are a constant reminder of the further potential psychological trauma of type 3. Perhaps this fact will suggest the emotional uneasiness which accompanies type 2 MS attacks.

With this brief introduction we now enter that strange world of ailments which are not apparent as belonging to MS to even a careful non-medical observer, but which usually are noted readily by highly trained specialists. In my case these symptoms have all been verified by both my physician and a specialist or a second physician. I was told in response to my inquiry each time that the problem was not hysterical and that there was a physical base, which I was to learn later was located in the central neural system.

Layered vision is one of the strange conditions that beset me. The event occurred in April 1962, three months after the myelogram. One day, toward noon, as I sat working in my office, my eyes began to bother me. It was a combination of lack of focus and a tiredness of the eyes which affected me. I was doing rather close work requiring great intellectual and visual attention. I had been working on a complex computer program for statistical analysis. The concentration required for this type of work cannot be sustained for many hours, and so I was not really surprised that it seemed like time for a break. As I relaxed in my chair, my vision came to rest on the doorknob across the office, a distance of perhaps fifteen to twenty feet. I saw not one but two knobs, and they persisted through various attempts to refocus my eyes and to rest them. I had double vision!

After perhaps a half-hour the problem was sufficiently distressing to move me to telephone for an early appointment with my physician. Fortunately his office hours were in the afternoon, and his nurse found time for me immediately. I must have walked the approximately three-quarters of a mile to his office, for we were then in our car-less period, a time which covered nearly the entire decade of the sixties. The physician confirmed my complaint by a series of examinations. Whatever he saw must have seemed important, for he made two referrals, one to our ophthalmologist and the second to the chairman of the department of neurology at Billings Hospital at The University of Chicago.

The ophthalmologist was our regular family eye-physician who had frequently examined my eyes. During this particular visit, however, she put me through an entirely different routine called "reading fields." I think the term "reading" here refers to her activity rather than mine, and the term "fields" stands for sections of a large wall chart. As I recall the chart, it was an extension of the various functions of the eye. You stared at the center of the chart and responded to questions about various colors and figures in different sections or fields of the chart. You were responding on the basis of partial rather than total eye function. In any event, this was an interesting and painless, though mysterious, procedure which led to reassurances and to the neurology clinic.

You should understand that at this point in time I did not know the diagnosis, nor was it to be revealed to me for nearly a decade. Moreover, it is not clear whether my physician had yet made the diagnosis, although he must have been highly suspicious. As best as I can reconstruct the events, this visit to the neurologist must have been the point at which the diagnosis was either made or confirmed. Once again the procedure was interesting and mysterious. The physician dealt with an extension of function, as the ophthalmologist had done. But extension of neural function can involve motion, so I found myself playing patty-cake and similar games with the neurologist's hands in various kinds of motion. Once again I was reassured by having the neurologist tell me that the double vision would go away after a little while. And it did, after about six weeks.

Toward the end of that period I entered my raccoon stage. The double vision had affected me sufficiently so that colleagues were aware of the difficulty. Many asked what it felt like. I found myself saying, and dramatizing with my hands, that it seemed as though there was more sensory input than I could handle. "It seems that if I could eliminate some of the peripheral vision I might be more comfortable. Perhaps if I had tunnel vision it would help." And I began to form peep-holes with my hands to demonstrate. Lo and behold, my vision did seem somewhat less confusing when looking through the peep-holes. So peep-hole glasses were created at home out of large sunglasses fitted with a paper cover on each lens, and a small hole prepared in each paper cover. This pair of glasses was worn for weeks until, as both the ophthalmologist and neurologist had said, the condition disappeared. My physician took some, but slight interest in the glasses. And though I am quite certain that they had nothing to do with the remission of that attack, the glasses did seem to reduce the distress of the double vision, perhaps by reducing the complexity of the field of vision which had to be perceived.

One of the strangest aspects of this particular symptom of MS is that I did not immediately recognize that the double vision was not ordinary, side-by-side double vision. Rather, the images appeared one slightly above the other in layers. In fact, only since learning of the general diagnosis of MS have I discovered that this particular kind of visual problem is known as layered vision.

In 1972 or 1973 the layered vision problem provided a very unique experience. We were having our bedroom carpeted with a medium length shag which was multi-colored like a tweed. Being interested in how carpeting is laid, I walked to the hallway and started the few steps necessary to reach the bedroom. The men had completed work near the doorway and were out of my sight, so my vision fell upon a floor full of this new, shaggy, multi-colored carpeting. The floor appeared to have been raised several inches, necessitating a step up to enter the room.

Instantly a conflict arose in my mind, for I knew the bedroom floor was level with the hall floor; yet clearly I was seeing a room with a raised floor. My vision was quickly averted from the room, for an irreconcilable conflict engrossed my mind. After several brief glimpses at the carpeted floor with ensuing consideration of the phenomenon, my composure returned. Whether during this transitory incident or later in the day I know not, but finally the illusion disappeared.

During late summer and early autumn of 1974, and at various times in 1975 and 1976, the layered vision popped up again in mild and temporary form. This leads me to believe that recurrence is dependent upon eye, or general, tiredness in addition to whatever else may be involved.

But let me not leave the topic of layered vision without reporting on its benefits. First, it makes you realize that there are physical grounds for believing that not everyone sees the world the same way. Perhaps artists do differ from other people in what and how they see, purely on a neurological basis. Second, some ordinary sights literally take on a new dimension when viewed with layered vision. Driving home one afternoon during the recurrence of the vision problem I suddenly found myself confronted by a large yellow sign, about a foot high, piled in the middle of the street. Fortunately it said "STOP," which I did. It took only a fraction of a second to realize that the size of the sign, the angle of vision, and my state of fatigue had converged to cause my layered vision to create a substantial three-dimensional stop sign out of a flat traffic order painted on the street. It literally loomed up from the street—that's weird.

Since that episode there have been occasions to check the double vision further. Late one winter afternoon as we drove east toward Michigan my double vision again became noticeable. The interrupted white line down the middle of the eastbound two lanes of a divided highway appeared much as had the three-dimensional stop sign. Each segment of the line tended to be reproduced slightly in front of the paint. This gave semblance of a three-dimensional divider. Having wondered more about the nature of this condition, I tried viewing the center line first through one eye, then the other, straddling the line with the car. The doubled, three-dimensional line appeared for each eye. It was offset slightly to the right when viewed through the left eye, and offset to the left for the right eye. Crosseyed double vision offers two objects side by side.

We turn our attention next to a sticky valve. Apparently several places in the human body are equipped with a ring of muscle which can act to close or open passages between organs or external body openings. Such a muscle is known as an annular muscle, and the tissue acted upon together with the muscle is called a sphincter. I have heard the particular one to be discussed here called the sphincter valve. Whether this name is respected among physicians I cannot say, but it is a suggestive name which will thus be used here.

The sphincter valve of concern is the one controlling the outlet from the bladder. Anyone who has visited any except the most fastidious of homes for elderly will recognize instantly that the odor of urine which permeates such homes is directly related to the sphincter valve. For many elderly persons the problem is no doubt a weakening of the muscle which operates to close the bladder.

Many persons with multiple sclerosis have continuing difficulty with this particular sphincter valve, not because of lowered muscle tone, as might well be the case with the elderly, but rather because messages directing the valve to close don't get through. More accurately, it seems, the message is often interrupted. This results in what has been labeled "the dribbles" and worse. Again, the difference between MS types 2 and 3 is substantial so far as this difficulty is concerned. A type 2 patient, if my experience is not unique, can manage to some extent with the exercise of patience and careful closing ceremony, so to speak. Caution in the form of preparedness is also necessary for those occasions when the valve seems on the verge of opening without seeking permission.

My wife and I can probably furnish an unbelievably long list of rest rooms in several cities in England and throughout Europe. The list could, no doubt, be subdivided for particular neighborhoods in London and Paris. For Chicago I could probably furnish direction to a men's room in every store in the Loop. But, as I started to say, phase 3 MS patients seem necessarily bound (no pun intended) to the catheter and leg bag if they are to do any traveling, even for a half day.

So in MS we often seem to have a cantankerous sphincter valve which tends to receive messages to "open," but to have a deaf ear for messages to "wait before opening." This problem is stated formally as "losing bladder and bowel retention," or incontinence. But this is only half the story, and, believe it or not, the half with the more manageable consequences, so far as bladder function is the concern.

This truth was learned while we were on a weekend trip to visit our mothers in Michigan. In fact, it was this episode or attack which finally convinced my physician to disclose the diagnosis of multiple sclerosis to me. We left Chicago just past midafternoon on a Friday for the two-and-a-half hour drive. Upon arrival I successfully directed the operation of the sphincter valve as one among many routine activities such as telephoning, eating, planning, reading and sleeping.

By midafternoon of Saturday it was becoming obvious

that my valve was not working, and had not opened for nearly twenty-four hours. Discomfort was mounting. A frenzied call to the local family physician brought an immediate response. I was provided a diaper made from a bath towel and taken to the emergency room of the hospital. There, as we waited perhaps an additional half-hour, it became painfully obvious that the sphincter valve was not going to open under my direction. The physician catheterized me and drained about 1300 cc. of fluid. Next he attached a fitting to the catheter so I could operate it myself, taped the entire mechanism so it would remain in place, and made an appointment to see me Monday morning.

During the Monday appointment he probed into the background of the episode and found me woefully lacking in information but with faith in my physician. He asserted that messages should have been telling the valve to open, and said they must not have been getting through. I could find no flaw in his comments. With a solemn promise from me to go immediately to my physician upon my return to Chicago, he released me still catheterized.

As promised, I headed for my physician's office and recounted the activity of the weekend. Upon due reflection he decatheterized me. with instructions to drink lots of water and to return the next day. Fortunately the sphincter valve worked properly and upon my return to the office everything seemed all right. After due reflection, my physician said, as previously reported, that perhaps it was time to talk about my problems. In fairly short order he then said: "For a long time we have suspected that you have multiple sclerosis." He acted as though this was a hard blow falling on me. In fact, my recollection is that before stating the diagnosis he had said, "This may come as a shock to you." My reaction may have disappointed him, for I had absolutely no idea what multiple sclerosis was; and he told me nothing. But that has all been recounted earlier. My point here is that the sticky valve was a disconcerting, at one point dangerous, and always mystifying, symptom of the condition finally revealed as MS.

A somewhat more straightforward condition was that which we shall call "stilt legs." Nearly everyone has a secret, perhaps unconscious, criterion which is invoked when selecting an article to be purchased. One may be attracted to toiletries by a scent, the shape of the dispenser, or even the color or design on the package. At one point in the post-World War II history of automobiles in this country the manufacturers discovered that they needed only to change color schemes from year to year in order to attract new buyers; expensive retooling was passé for a time. Furniture, it seems, is often selected for purchase on the basis of the colors or pattern of the upholstery material, or even because material of a particular texture has been used. Advertising agencies are well aware of these facts.

If multiple sclerosis were a desirable commodity available on the open market, perhaps the most popular criterion in a decision whether or not to have it would be the quality of the leg affliction that goes with it. In such circumstance, I would have an advantage on the market, after hovering near type 3 MS for uncounted months. The phenomenon which I have since learned to respect as an attack struck with bewildering effect I know not when. Most certainly I moved on numbed legs almost continuously from the summer of 1971 until some time in 1973; but let me defer comment on that period until later, focusing here on the nature of the numbness.

Having had the sensation of legs wearing out in a mild form many times before, it is probable that the trauma was lessened, or perhaps easier to contemplate than it would have been had a pair of severely numbed legs occurred suddenly as a new sensation. Even so, I recall sitting dejectedly on the examining table, weeping and saying to my physician: "Go take care of your other patients; they are sick. There is nothing wrong with me." This episode must have unfolded some weeks or months after the onset of the numbness, for I recall having pointed out to him that I was beginning to wear my right shoe sole thin more quickly than the left shoe sole. As always he was noncommittal, and I wondered whether even such physical evidence of a medical problem might in fact point to a psychological cause. Such musings were extremely difficult to handle.

Considering more carefully the nature of the attack, two points seem clear: first, a paradox involving both numbness and hypersensitivity was involved; second, sensory nerve messages were affected more certainly than were motor nerve messages. The first of these two conditions qualifies the attack involving the legs as a weird wonderment. The fact that the second condition is not quite accurately stated, although basically true, adds to the strangeness to be considered.

Characterization of this attack of multiple sclerosis affecting the legs as "stilt legs" is suggested as not pure fantasy. Walking on stilts, as I remember from my youth, creates two challenges to the sensory system. On the one hand, the wooden extension of legs, which stilts are, have no neurological connection to the human system. They do, however, transmit vibrations as they strike the pavement. This enables the somatic sensory system to act as a kinesthetic nervous system, taking cues from positions of the feet and legs as well as the amplitude of the sound vibration emanating from the end of the stilts as they strike and scrape the pavement. On the other hand, balance is difficult to maintain, not because there is anything basically wrong with the intricate balancing system, but because you have no direct control over the stilts, directing them only second-handedly, so to speak. This requires some anticipation of corrective action, but even that cannot obliterate some of the lurching, unsteady activity which almost necessarily accompanies stilt-walking.

The stilt leg symptoms of type 2 required adjustments in order to carry on a reasonably normal-appearing life. Fortunately we were still in our car-less years when the attack struck so that driving was not a problem. By the time we had again become owners of an automobile there still seemed to be no problem in handling the vehicle safely. Whether this was because of learning how to handle the numb legs over time, or because the severity of the attack had lessened, or because extended caution was exercised in providing margins for error, I do not know.

Walking, however, was a challenge and I learned to appreciate Archibald MacLeish's lines:

> The labor of order has not rest:
> To impose on the confused, fortuitous
> Flowing away of the world, Form—
> Still, cool, clean, obdurate,
>
> Lasting forever, or at least
> Lasting: a precarious monument
> Promising immortality, for the wing
> Moves and in the moving balances.

Diane wrote the MacLeish in the front of a book on existential philosophy and sent it from Paris as a birthday gift to "my daddy" in 1969. I have treasured that gift, particularly the poem, and have refrained from asking about it. It resonated richly within my experience; one could hardly ask more.

Motion in a natural gait, befitting my height and stride, was the easiest mode of behavior to control, perhaps because habit took command. Somehow standing still seemed to deprive me of sensory information needed to remain upright. Some swaying, shifting of weight, and shuffling of feet were used to provide partial kinesthetic information. Such attempted substitution of activity for more natural movement was less than satisfactory. Not only was the substitute motion less aesthetically pleasing, it also failed to provide the range of kinesthetic information normally monitored by an upright person in natural motion.

From time to time a severely afflicted man walks from home to work in my neighborhood, a distance of approximately one mile. From the random set of times he has come into my view it seems likely that he walks both to and from work several days each week in many kinds of weather. His affliction is unknown to me but both spinal malformation and a type of motor discoordination seem involved. His normal posture is bent forward from the hips at a severe angle. To see him standing or sitting with his cane is to wonder how he could walk. But underway he moves in an amazing array of continuous, unusual motions which enable him to get where he intends to go ". . . for the wing moves and in the moving balances."

One does learn to look down while walking on numbed legs. As an acquaintance with MS joked, "I certainly find a lot of money on the ground now that I look down while walking." Failure to attend to the path you are about to tread is disciplined vigorously by stumbles over half-inch rises in sidewalk seams and forward lunges as your feet rise not quite high enough while you climb stairs. In winter I learned to grasp railings in subways, department stores, train stations, office buildings—wherever ascent or descent was required. When outside temperatures no longer required that gloves be worn, the textures, state of repair, and state of cleanliness of railings invited me to learn a trick. This was to keep one hand in a constant state of readiness, poised about an inch above or below railings and prepared to grasp instantly should sensory misjudgment cause a misstep threatening a headlong descent of a subway stair. Practice can lead to a triumphant sense of accomplishment, but one must be mindful not to become proud.

Of course the degree of stilt-leggedness which separates MS types 2 and 3 is not distinct. Some acquaintances who share a type 2 diagnosis are able to walk only with the aid of a cane or other support, and then only with great effort at times. But clearly they are ambulatory, and patients with a phase 3 diagnosis are not. Furthermore, ambulatory patients with more severe leg symptoms than mine are often fiercely determined to remain self-sufficient in this regard. Having fallen in their homes they may take five, ten, even fifteen minutes to get up again, but they do rise and walk on.

Occasional tiredness in the knees today floods the mind with visual images, both recalled and fantasied, of persons collapsing and stumbling. It also reminds me of the Cleveland attack which, you may recall, struck a nerve which wended its way from the spine to the knee and seemed to disappear in or under the kneecap. At that time no symptom of fatigue or inoperativeness was apparent. During the period of stilt-leggedness, fatigue in the legs was not a factor so far as I could determine. Walking problems were attributed to lack of good and accurate information getting through the nervous system. One wonders, without really wanting to find out personally, what amount or combination of sensory input and muscle-directing output is involved in the gradations of affliction of the legs between types 2 and 3 of multiple sclerosis.

Among the memories from my history of attacks of MS are several which exemplify the paradox of simultaneous numbness and hypersensitivity. Perhaps these should be labeled "hypersensitive numbness." Examples are sprinkled through the chapters to come, but the sticky valve discussed earlier in this chapter is a useful introduction to the topic. The hypersensitivity part of the paradox of the bladder sphincter is, upon analysis, probably manifested by what is called "nervous bladder."

Without providing details, it can be explained as based on a muscle with nerves which ordinarily sense a distended bladder and signal a need for relief. This signal is probably dual, that is, it probably is sent to two places: to a conditioned reflex which needs a second, confirming signal from, perhaps, the brain; and to the brain which in turn sets off the reflex by adding its confirming message. The nervous bladder seems to send messages to the brain much too soon so the person thinks he has a full bladder when he hasn't. Without the initial, direct message from the sensing muscle, the valve won't open. But persistent, conscious efforts by the person to obey the false message from the bladder result in a successful "willing" of the sphincter to open. But operating on only a persistent half of the required pair of messages, the valve soon closes, resulting in what my physician calls "difficulty in starting and stopping" or "dribbling."

Living with this kind of hypersensitivity sets you up for the time when the nerve in the sensing muscle sends both messages but numbness or a short-circuit prevents either the direct message to the valve or the brain-mediated message from being received. Willing does not succeed in this case and the only solution is the catheter.

The episode involving both hypersensitivity and numbness in the legs and in one arm and hand are recounted elsewhere. Fatigue, reflexes in the feet, and depression will be discussed later and mentioned in connection with the paradox of hypersensitivity and numbness. At this time I should like to describe and discuss a phenomenon which is categorizable as a manifestation of hypersensitivity. This discussion is an effort to suggest that I am not talking about a little tickle under the chin when discussing hypersensitivity. The focal point was my right ear.

At some point there developed a mild sensation of itching in my right ear. My physician examined the ear and found nothing foreign in it. Taking into account the possibility that some tiny foreign body might have intruded deep into the ear, he flushed it, perhaps more than once, with tepid water. The itching sensation persisted on an intermittent schedule and I informed him of this during my next appointment. He looked again and asked me if I didn't mean to report that the left ear bothered me. He thought the left ear seemed more suspicious than the right. I think he said to let him know if things didn't get better. They didn't and I did let him know. But this time I had a foul cold in the head. He referred me to the ENT specialist in the clinic, saying to him, "But you've got to take this other thing into account, too." I thought that a dark saying since I had been informed of no "other thing," but the occasion passed with no further illumination on that saying. It was one of many odd sentences which were to be cleared up when I learned that MS had struck me.

The ENT man sorted things out quickly, treating me for the nose and throat involvement in the cold, and prescribing a fluid to be dropped into the right ear two or three times each day. His advice to keep *everything* else, including water, out of the ear for the time being suggests that an appropriate designation of this episode might be "the little boy's delight." I was to be advised to keep water out of that ear for a period of about three years.

After faithfully conforming to the ENT physician's plan of treatment, I returned to his office for an appointment a few weeks later. The cold symptoms had disappeared but the ear problem persisted. A continuation of the eardrops was recommended, and a refillable prescription for the drops was given to me. The drops were continued until different advice was received.

My first contact with the ENT physican was made in November. The following November I made an appointment with an ear specialist at a center for medical research, for the condition had worsened to the point of being nearly unbearable.

From the beginning this condition seemed like an itch deep in the right ear, but it became a "heavier" sensation. It seemed as though scratching would not relieve the sensation even if the itching point could be reached. Then the sensation spread upward and outward on the ear. Sometimes it seemed as if the ear had been invaded by tiny bugs which marched out of the ear along several paths which radiated like a spider web. As they marched they irritated the ear along these radiating paths. Nothing was very effective in stopping the problem. The drops prescribed by the first ENT physician were useless. No amount of covering, scratching or rubbing ever reduced the sensation or caused it to stop. One morning, while riding in an elevated train, the sensation spread to the scalp area around the ear. It was also throbbing or pulsating. Vividly do I recall almost huddling in the seat, knowing not what to do for relief. Eventually a shudder ran through my body. Further than that my memory of that episode is blank. However, it seems to me that from that time forward I was aware of two characteristics of this phenomenon. One was the throbbing of the network area. The second characteristic was the schedule of occurrence. I never paid sufficient attention to the times of onset to be able to chart them, but they seemed to be on some kind of schedule. Part of that schedule was the duration of the feeling once it started. It appeared to recede or fade after an hour or two.

The intensity of sensation in and around my right ear, and the obvious lack of effectiveness of treatment by the first ENT physician, drove me to the examining room of the ear specialist. He said he found a severe infection of the eardrum. After cleaning the drum as best he could he had me discard the original eardrops and he prescribed a different kind of drops with an oil base. He said the new drops would leave no residue; the old ones did and in fact may have contributed to the infection.

Before explaining the probable connection of this ailment to MS, I should like to share the wonders of a trip to the office of a modern specialist on ears. Two procedures are of particular interest. The first must have some purpose, but it has never been clear to me. It consists of having the patient inhale and hold his breath. The physician counts to some specified number, perhaps it was 3. On the count of three the patient holds his breath. At the exact instant the patient starts to hold in air on the count of 3, the physician blows mightily through a tube he has inserted into your mouth. The eardrums and eyeballs must have distended a foot!

The second notable procedure was having your ear vacuum cleaned. Yes, vacuum cleaned! This otolaryngologist had an extensive set of beautiful miniature instruments, one of which was a tiny vacuum cleaner, tank type. He inserted the nozzle and tube into the ear and, while peering into the ear, he vacuumed it. Once or twice the eardrum was sucked up tightly against the nozzle causing slight pain, but in general this was an interesting and painless procedure.

This physician's instructions were to use the oil-based drops morning and evening and to keep everything else, including water, out of the ear. He called the condition by some name which did not register with me. The severity of the itching and throbbing diminished but did not disappear. Within a few weeks the physician reported that the infection had cleared, but the original problem persisted. Whether this physician knew of my diagnosis I do not know. Since the original diagnosis, or confirmation, had been made many years earlier at these same clinics, it is conceivable but not certain that he saw the old records. In any event he permitted me to continue using the ear drops for a couple of years after the infection disappeared. It was never clear to me whether or not the drops had an effect on the itching, but it seemed as though they might, and so the drops were continued.

During the course of treatment for the ear infection the physician once said, "The wax is beginning to come back; that's good." Then I realized that the right ear had not been yielding wax as had the left ear. It did not yield a normal quantity until the original complaint of itching disappeared.

It was during this ear episode that my physician revealed my condition to me. The more I read and wondered, the more clearly it seemed that the ear problem had been three-fold. One problem had been infection; this was probably not related to MS. But the itching, throbbing ear was probably a derivative of the hypersensitivity occasioned by MS. And the wax shutdown was probably caused by disturbance of a nerve, again caused by MS. The itching seemed to belong to the same category as other hypersensitivity conditions related elsewhere. The lack of wax involved a gland, and fits in the category with a gallbladder attack and consequent gastro-intestinal problems; they could all stem from an attack on the visceral nerve system. Some day I shall ask the otolaryngologist whether or not he knew of my basic health problem. If not, he is entitled to know, for it seems to explain the persistence of some symptoms after the ear infection had cleared.

One other recurring symptom seems appropriately classified in the series of weird happenings which have marked the course of my MS. This particular symptom may be related to lightheadedness, but it seems like a distinct, independent symptom to me. I call it "thinking down a barrel."

If you have ever called into a cistern, tried to make a jug or a barrel resonate with your voice, or yelled into a long pipe, you may have some idea of what I am trying to convey about thinking down a barrel. One characteristic of sound in a large chamber is that it gets lost for there is not enough of it to fill the chamber, except perhaps for a fleeting moment. Even that moment is dependent upon your creating a sound consonant with the natural overtone series of the chamber.

Another characteristic of your voice projected into a cistern, pipe, or barrel is that it no longer sounds very much like your voice. Almost any voice, if tuned to the chamber, will resound in such manner that the chamber, rather than the person, seems to be creating the sound.

Yet another characteristic of cisterns, barrels, and the like is that they seem to make your voice come from a distance. It is almost as though you were listening and hearing another voice, perhaps coming from the bottom of the well.

So perhaps you can imagine what I mean by "thinking down a barrel." Your thought seems too small to fill whatever it is you are thinking in. There is no way to momentarily fill the chamber with thought, for resonance does not seem characteristic of thought. The thoughts in a barrel seem distant, perhaps not yours. This experience is of the same order as the experience of living through a situation which you feel to have been in before. You easily, accurately, and eerily forecast every action and predict every utterance. The similarity to "thinking down a barrel" resides in the fact that both have the distant, detached quality. If you have never experienced either of these phenomena you will probably not have the slightest idea what is being suggested. If your lot is to have avoided such events,

I know not whether to pity or congratulate you. The experiences are very interesting though somewhat upsetting. It can be said with assurance, however, that if "thinking down a barrel" has some form of MS as a prerequisite, best forget it. Interesting as such thinking is, it is not worth the impairment to the central nervous system which is implied by MS.

In concluding this chapter on strange, even weird, events in the progress of my attacks of MS, let us turn again to the consideration made at the beginning of the chapter. The first point to be made was that this group of symptoms ranged widely over the functions affected. We have seen an affliction of eyesight in the form of layered vision. And by the way, this common symptom is sometimes outdone by episodes of blindness in MS patients. Mine has been the good fortune to have avoided even temporary blindness.

A second symptom, a sticky valve, took us to the bladder region where signals to the sphincter are necessary if it is to open and close properly.

Stilt legs focused attention on symptomatic problems from the hips to the toes. This condition is also seen as variable across MS types 2 and 3.

The ear problems returned our considerations to the cranial end of the patient, and the thoughts in a barrel may have moved us completely out of the skull.

Overriding these various ailments is the paradoxical set of conditions of numbness and hypersensitivity. One or the other of these conditions seems to accompany most symptoms of MS.

I suggest that this is an array of weird symptoms. Let me suggest further that when you are afflicted by them you begin to wonder what is happening to you.

Next we move to some of the more conventional complaints of MS patients.

6

Conventional Complaints

Even though it may be true that each MS patient has a different pattern of complaints and ailments, there are, nevertheless, many standard complaints. In fact, patients with MS report being astounded to hear the chief neurologist at an MS clinic recite some of their problems when they first appear at the clinic after a prior diagnosis elsewhere. Let me not imply that the neurologist always does this, for such behavior would constitute an inappropriate practice for a physician. But there are enough conventional complaints to enable a specialist in MS to make the recitation suggested above.

Figures from various studies indicate that two symptoms head the list of neurological signs evident in MS. The absence of abdominal reflexes and the presence of the reflex which extends your foot when stimulated on the sole occur in 80 to 90 per cent of MS cases. These are followed by wiggly-eyed nystagmus (involuntary rapid eyeball movement), with roughly a 70 to 80 per cent incidence, impaired vibratory sensing, and impaired postural sensing, with weakness of lower limbs occurring in an average of about half the cases. Many more symptoms could be added to the list, but the per cent of cases in which they occur drops off to less than fifty.

The list of initial symptoms of MS is different from the list of symptoms occurring in the highest percentage of cases. Weaknesses tops the list of symptoms at the beginning of MS, scoring near 50 per cent. Some kind of visual problem, double vision or blurred vision, is the next most frequent initial symptom. Ataxia, or impaired coordination, is the third most frequent initial symptom, followed by paresthesia, which is a tickling or a burning sensation on the skin.

Earlier we have discussed numbness, layered vision, fatigue, bladder malfunction, itchy ear, and loss of feeling in the legs. These are all candidates for the conventional complaints department even though they have characteristics which set them apart from other standard symptoms. Some of the less exotic, standard problems which will be discussed here are: bumping, lightheadedness, aggression, fatigue, inability to focus attention, false bladder signals, and loss of memory for words. If this sounds like a recitation of unrelated problems, you are perhaps developing some sense of the nature of MS as experienced by the patient. As my physician said relatively early in my case, "You certainly do spread your ailments around."

But it is not the diversity of problems which is the focus here, although the diversity is a factor which affects you psychologically. Rather, the intent here is to attempt to convey the nature of some of the more commonly heard complaints as well as to stress the constancy with which a particular problem forces itself upon your attention. Some instances are comical, perhaps even the entire syndrome of consequences of a symptom are humorous, but they are,

nonetheless, demanding intruders on the stream of consciousness.

For example, consider the problem that could be
called "bumping." Stated baldly, it is the problem of knock-
ing into things: perhaps you fail to lift the juice glass high
enough to clear the coffee cup; sometimes you bump the
slice of bread against the toaster as you prepare to toast
it; or you fail to negotiate a doorway, slamming an arm or
shoulder against the frame as you start to move through.
As I sit here writing there are two small scarred areas on
the back of my right hand, reminders of recent clumsiness.

Bumping can make one a firm believer in witchcraft.
How else can you explain the shrunken doorways, now
marred through efforts to move chairs from one room to
another? Before the doorways shrank, the furniture could
be moved readily through the openings. And what other
than witchcraft could transform a davenport or chair into
a football player prepared to block you at thigh height
when you attempt to walk around one of its corners? Perhaps the most annoying, though clever manifestation of
witchcraft, is making you think you have turned right or
left when, in fact, only your body has started to change
direction. Your feet are still moving in the original direction. If not bruised too badly, you can at times see the
humor in the situation. Comics have entertained through
centuries, no doubt, with sight gags based on bumps of this
kind.

The orange juice spilling type of problem is probably
the result of an improperly calculated fine adjustment of
the muscles. You lift the glass high all right, but you fail to
lift it quite high enough, either because some needed information did not reach the processing center, or the proper
signal failed to reach the muscles. The failure to turn when
you think you have turned is, no doubt, a straight-forward

failure of any signal to reach the legs. Often the body trunk will have twisted slightly in the desired direction. Whatever the explanation, when an attack with these symptoms strikes, it cannot be ignored; there are simply too many daily occasions which involve potential bumping for it to be put out of mind easily or for very long.

The same thing can happen to hands, feet, knees, elbows, arms, legs, and heads. They can all be bumped mildly or severely as a result of improperly controlled messages which move them, for MS interferes with message control in the central nervous system. Part of the bumping phenomenon would appear to be associated with a slowed transmission of information to the legs. If, as has been stated, heavily myelinated nerve fibers conduct impulses more rapidly than those with a thin or slim myelin cover, then any loss of myelin from nerves to the legs might act to reduce the speed of messages to the legs. Something like this must occur when I find my shoulder against a doorframe, partially headed in a new direction, and my feet still pointed in my previously intended direction.

Another common complaint among MS patients who are still mobile is lightheadedness. Unfortunately, lightheadedness seems to be used to cover several undifferentiated conditions, which makes both their diagnosis and management difficult. Possibly there is no management which can be applied to this syndrome. One symptom available only to the patient is simple lightheadedness. I am unable to describe it other than to say that it seems like a ring applied to the head as an ascending or lifting series of circles, sometimes visualized, often in colors. At times lightheadedness is accompanied by one or another sensation involving the ears; one time the sensation may be a ringing, another time it seems as though the ears had been unstopped, not unlike the earpopping when changing air pressure aboard an aircraft. Typically little or no feeling of faintness is felt.

Sometimes the lightheadedness is more certainly dizziness and can undoubtedly be traced to having messages from the inner ear distorted or delayed. Looking upward quickly, perhaps toward the top of skyscrapers or at airborne objects nearly overhead, will result in this kind of dizziness. But there is yet another kind of lightheadedness. This type, known as nystagmus, is a dizziness caused by irregular motion of the eyes. It has been said to be the most common of all the symptoms of multiple sclerosis.

Nystagmus is not dizziness; rather it is an apparently natural set of eye movements designed to help avoid dizziness. Here we have another of the paradoxes of MS. If you have ever watched a tap or ballet dancer or a free-style ice-skater you have seen attempts to apply the idea of nystagmus to movement of the head. These performers do not allow their heads to whirl as their bodies do. If you watch closely, the head seems to face toward some object until the whirl is about half completed. At this point the head is jerked around more rapidly than the body so it again faces the same object. This is vaguely analogous to the eye movements involved in nystagmus. When you turn, your eyes receive signals from the inner ear. They focus on an object momentarily then jump to another object and so on throughout the turn. The problem which often arises from MS is that on occasion something causes the eyes to act as though you were in motion even though you are not. The eyes drift sideways then jerk back to the original position, eventually causing dizziness. This paradox is also hard to ignore when it arises.

If you will forgive an aside, let me dwell for a moment on the topic eyes. They seem to hold an immense fascination for physicians. Annual checkups always include having the physician peer through his ophthalmoscope into first one then the other eye. The only physician among the many who have examined me who chose not to examine my eyes was the one who ran the myelogram show. The delicate tissue inside the eye enables the physician to estimate the condition of the blood vessels and who knows what else. Perhaps Kay's ophthalmologist carried the art of interpreting the eyeball to the pinnacle recently. As she gazed into the interior of one eye, she said to Kay, "You must have been a towhead when you were young. You must have been very light complexioned." I wonder how reading eyeballs ever escaped becoming a parlor game.

Next we turn to aggression, a topic which is controversial, at least among patients with type 2 MS. First off, aggression is defined as "unprovoked attack." Few, if any acquaintances with MS would admit to launching any kind of "unprovoked attack," be it verbal or physical. They do agree that a heightened state of sensitivity makes them irritable and thus perhaps liable to overestimate the degree of provocation to which they are being subjected. That is to say their threshold of tolerance is lowered so that a casual observer might think he was witnessing an unprovoked attack.

But this is not the only difficulty encountered when the MS patient considers aggression. There is a tendency for those who know the patient's diagnosis to suggest that he is "using" MS to rationalize behavior about a problem quite independent of the condition. For example, mother-in-law problems, problems with children (of any age), rip-offs by the mechanic or his boss at the garage, drivers who endanger your vehicle if not your life or limb in heavy traffic, bait-and-switch tactics in many businesses, false advertising—all of these are candidates for generating aggression among the most staid of citizens. When an MS patient suggests that his condition renders him hypersensitive to such provocations, the listener often suggests that MS is only being used to rationalize aggressiveness in the individual.

MS patients seem to be supportive of one another's aggression saying that a particular aggressive act is justified and not merely the reaction of a hypersensitive person. I recall my father's story of the patient man and the dishonest butcher. The butcher, when weighing meat, was skillful at laying his thumb gently on the scale platform while both he and the customer gazed intently at the weight indicator. One day the man's patience was exhausted. He stepped behind the counter, grasped a meat cleaver and ordered the butcher to place his thumb on the block. The surprised butcher asked what the man had in mind. Replied he, "I've bought that thumb every week for years. Today I'm taking it home with me."

One young married mother we know is afflicted with MS which is in between types 2 and 3. She once related what she would like to say to her insistent mother-in-law: "Look, I'm just too tired to go shopping with you today. I'm sorry!" She feared, however, that she would be using her condition as an excuse to escape from a routine she didn't enjoy and acting aggressively at the same time. Her acquaintances, after probing a bit into her degree of tiredness, assured her that her fears were not well-founded, that it would be appropriate to be both honest and firm with her mother-in-law about this matter. But one can see, perhaps, that aggression does create dilemmas, which in turn can create nagging feelings of guilt.

If you were to think that the symptoms of MS enumerated up to this point, both conventional and odd, should leave the patient tired, you would be on the right track but far from the station. He is exhausted, or easily becomes so. This symptom, not entirely a reflection of other symptoms, is known not surprisingly as fatigue. The source of fatigue, or rather its cause, is apparently not really known. A computer engineer, the husband of an acquaintance with MS, was impressed when a neurologist discussed the central nervous system in terms of wires, electrical impulses, telephone cables, switchboards, etc. The engineer later said that perhaps our fatigue was due to the short-circuiting of nerves. He suggested that a lot of power could be dissipated through a short-circuit, especially if there were no fuse to interrupt the flow of energy. This suggests a neurological explanation of fatigue. Yet another possibility is that the cause of fatigue is depression. Just how depression is defined is not clear in the material I have read, but the idea seems valid to me. This might be a good point for chemopsychiatrists to focus on; they could be guaranteed a large supply of experimental subjects from the ranks of MS patients.

Yet another view of fatigue suggests that it arises from the excessive expenditure of muscular energy. The tricky word here is "excessive," for it is defined as energy expenditure which is fatiguing. But circularity aside, multiple sclerosis does reduce the amount of energy available before fatigue sets in. How energy is reduced is not clear, but that a smaller amount of physical exertion is required to induce fatigue in MS patients than in "normal" people is clear.

What is fatigue like? What are its characteristics? Not surprisingly one characteristic is physical tiredness bordering on exhaustion. Most of us have been near exhaustion from some activity we enjoy, such as playing ball at a picnic, building things for the children's play yard, pouring a cement patio, or hiking and climbing. Exhaustion from such activities usually is accompanied by a good feeling, a feeling of satisfaction, perhaps enhanced by the realization that you were able to accomplish the challenging activity. Fatigue in the condition of MS is not like that; it is not lightened or eased by the sense of accomplishment.

As I have suggested over and over, strange, even para-doxical things transpire in MS, and such is the case with fatigue. The ego-supporting thought of accomplishment which can relieve physical fatigue doesn't just fail to act, its absence seems to trigger a reaction which deepens the fatigue in MS. Psychological fatigue, due partially to occa-sional overwork of the sensory nerves, adds to the con-dition, deepening the fatigue. In my case, with the diagnosis concealed from me, the further burden of wondering whether some of the problems encountered might be psychosomatic drove me to the edge of despair at one point. The situation during which this state was reached, an office call, will be reported in Chapter IX. None of my conversations with other patients has been in sufficient depth to enable me to infer with great certainty that they too had confronted despair, but it would be surprising if despair were not a characteristic experience for persons with type 2 symptoms or beyond.

With MS one sleeps nine or ten hours, occasionally uninterrupted, even when one has performed precious little physical work, and only slightly more productive mental work. Of course, "occasionally uninterrupted" means on those rare occasions when you are not awakened by false bladder signals or jerky legs, etc. But the most insidious characteristic of my fatigue was an increasing inability to focus on a task long enough to complete it. There is more said about attention span in the next chapter, but here it seems appropriate to mention some activities which might have resulted from either fatigue or a short attention span.

As clear an example as I know of inability to focus attention on a task is the following episode involving a re-search project. In 1965 I undertook a project which in-volved applying some ideas from information theory to some data on reading. The data were all gathered within a period of about a year. This left three tasks to be completed: a conventional analysis of the data, a second analysis using ideas from information theory, and a summarization of the two analyses indicating what the ideas from information theory suggested about reading which were new and different from the conventional analysis. Although these tasks were turned to time and again, the net result was that the work from these uncompleted tasks was merely piled upon or beside other incomplete work. Finally, after about eight years, the work was finished. It should have been completed within two years of the time the first data were gathered. This episode occurred in the midst of my encounters with the unknown antagonist, MS.

Another sign of my lack of focus and energy was the top of my desk. Prior to the second half of the 1960's it had been customary to clear my desk completely by the end of August each year. As of early 1975, the complete top of my desk had not been visible in eleven years. Various kinds of mail, odd assortments of bibliographies for potential projects, unfinished manuscripts and assorted other items filled the desktop and the tops of my file cabinets. Some improvement is now visible. An acquaintance once had such a scene straightened and made neat by a secretary who wanted to surprise him. His anger was nearly unbridled as he pointed to the cleared, clean, dustless object and said, "There was a certain amount of information in the way things were piled on that desk." I cannot make the same claim. My only excuse has been inability to focus my energies to any significant degree over a long period of years. Also, of course, the energy available for focusing was limited. It is my earnest hope that the recent, slight improvement may continue, even accelerate.

Recently Kay and I attended the thirty-fifth anniversary party for our high school class. One of the class members, we will call her Carol, attended with her husband. She came to the dinner unaccompanied, stating that her husband would appear soon. I asked what he looked like so as to be able to locate and guide him to the banquet room. She said, "Oh he's kind of fat." When I found him, he did not seem fat to me. In my view he was a good-looking, trim, well-dressed man. I wondered whether Carol was associating "lazy", which she later used as a synonym for lack of energy, with the word "fat." Somehow Kay had remembered that Carol's husband was stricken by MS, although his symptoms were undetectable that evening. Later Carol and I chatted at some length.

She and her husband had just moved from a city to an almost rural suburban area. Carol was becoming increasingly dissatisfied for there was a great deal of work to be done. Further, her husband wasn't doing many of the things which most husbands do, such as mowing the grass and keeping things in repair around the house. She complained that he didn't appear to have anything wrong with himself. She even hinted that he might be a bit lazy. Her dissatisfaction was apparent, as was her assumption that there was nothing wrong with him. Kay had told Carol that I too had MS. That was one of the reasons for our chatting. I told her of some of my symptoms and problems including fatigue. She was urged to judge her husband with understanding, although this would not relieve her of the extra chores she now performs. She was also urged to investigate an MS center where they might attend group discussion sessions, and explore what it means to have MS or to have a spouse with MS.

This event is reported in an effort to suggest how insidious MS fatigue is. How can any healthy-looking adult man be so tired when he does so little? Don't try it. You might be unpleasantly surprised.

It is odd that certain events remain in your memory, even some which lasted but a second or two. Such an event often is an insight. Gestalt theory in psychology would have us use such events as the basis for instructing, but in my ex-perience such insights are too widely scattered to be of much value in any curriculum which calls for planned in-struction over an extended subject matter. Nonetheless, one of the flashes of insight which I recall is relevant to the discussion of fatigue. One spring day while climbing the stairs to the third floor of our office building, I suddenly realized that it was easier to do than it had been for a long time. Suddenly there seemed to be more energy available. Then I realized that the level of energy at that moment was not extraordinary, that it was about what could be called normal for me. If so, then I had been operating on a significantly reduced level of energy for per-haps a couple of years. This event was but another of my mid-1960 experiences. Unfortunately, the return of a high level of energy at that time was shortlived.

The fact that one realizes he has lost something only upon regaining it may very well be an event in the psycho-logical realm more often than in the physical. Such an event is certainly an arresting one when it happens. Our daughter was once head nurse on a burn unit in a metropolitan hos-pital. Some months after leaving the job to raise a family she said to her mother, "I have regained my sense of humor. I had no idea I had lost it until it started coming back."

Returning for the moment to the discussion of fatigue, let me report that MS patients say they have infallible early warning of fatigue. Each patient seems to have a unique cue that further activity should be curtailed. For some it is a feeling in a limb or a joint, for others a slight head- or backache. In my case the early warning sign was an incom-plete belt of pain near the top of my hips. When the pain began, it was necessary for me to get off my feet. Pre-viously I had started to say that an early warning sign was a choice point, but that is not true. At least in my case, once the pain started it would not subside until some more restful activity or pose were begun. In fact, the pain heightened if rest were not sought.

After several years of visitation by the belt of pain, I decided to try to counter it. Since the sensation was something like being slowly strangled around the waist, the countering measure, I discovered, was to inhale deeply and then to press the air downward. This turned out to yield a period of very effective temporary relief, permitting me to extend for perhaps a half hour the bearable period of standing. Of course the breathing trick had to be repeated quite often, but an additional half hour is sometimes all that is needed to finish selective viewing in an art gallery or museum, or to get one back to the restaurant area of a zoo, or to complete shopping in a particular department store.

Eventually the band of pain around my waist, my personal indicator of the limit of my endurance, disappeared. Later, perhaps in 1974, a new sensation arose in the hip area. It felt like quite a different pain from what had seemed previously to be a muscle pain. It did not yield to the exercise of pressing downward thus forcing the abdomen outward against the offending muscle. It also appeared at a different time, during the night and early morning rather than during the day when I was active on my feet. Both my family physician and Dr. Davis at the MS Center informed me that it was "a touch of arthritis." A common pain reliever was prescribed. This seems not to have been an isolated incident in my web of odd symptoms.

When an occasional patient with severe arthritis appeared at the MS camp I wondered why. A range of debilitating conditions was evident among the campers, but arthritis was puzzling. Why should arthritis patients attend this camp? I never asked. But I did discover that rheumatoid arthritis is believed to be a so-called autoimmune disease in which the body's defense mechanisms go awry.

From one point of view, then, MS and arthritis, at least rheumatoid arthritis, are believed to belong to the same category of disease. This imperfect knowledge, valid or not, seemed to make my new pain less mysterious, although not diminished. Even the world of disease, it seems, is a small one.

Those who fail to heed the early warning signal report finding themselves in awkward situations. For example, one acquaintance is in the habit of walking several blocks to the train after work. He walks with determination, though his pace is less than brisk. On occasion his early warning cue suggests that he forego the walk and catch a cab. Being a creature of habit as well as bullheaded, he sometimes ignores the signal and attempts the walk. Typically this leads him to a seat on the steps of a building along the way, garnering and husbanding enough energy to hail and skirmish for a cab, when an empty one happens along.

Hypersensitivity is one of the characteristic conditions endured by MS patients. Here the reference is not to psychological hypersensitivity, which is also a burden, but rather to physical hypersensitivity. Frankly I must admit that sometimes one wonders whether a particular episode really is physical in nature. For example, there were times when I felt as though someone were sandpapering my nerves over a wide area of the nervous system. This is not more bearable after you learn that you have MS, although it may be more avoidable. Keeping the body temperature from rising is for me a first-class method for avoiding the general sandpapering effect. But rising temperature can be both physically and psychologically based.

Upon occasion there are somewhat less severe degrees of the condition known as hypersensitivity. I have previously mentioned that at one time my physician was endangered whenever he touched my feet. The reflexes in them seemed to be both highly sensitive and extremely vigorous. In the ear episode the region around and in the ear was very sensitive in an irritating way.

There were two other episodes characterized by apparent hypersensitivity. One involved the back of my head and the back of my neck. A great deal of time was spent scratching and rubbing these areas. The cartoon strip character named Itchy, who was forever scratching himself one place or another, came to mind. The second location which more than once was affected by the itching manifestation of hypersensitivity was the shoulder blade and upper chest area; the top of the trunk might be an accurate characterization. Again, there seemed to be no relief, you just scratched and rubbed. After having learned the nature of my basic condition, the itching problem became an intellectual problem too. The likelihood was that the itch was not located where it seemed to be. Rather, it was probably a feeling emanating from a tiny section of demyelinated nerve far distant from the point of discomfort. Should you scratch or rub? Whether or not you should, it is clear that you do. I am thankful that some of the episodes of hypersensitivity were of short duration, lasting perhaps a few days. Others, as you have seen, have lasted several years.

Let me try once again to impress you with the paradoxes attendant to MS by shifting from hypersensitivity back to numbness for a moment. The situation has been captured by a photograph of a bride-to-be standing arm-in-arm with her father just as they were about to proceed to the altar. It is, of course, our daughter's wedding and I am apparently deep in thought. Everyone enjoys suggesting what father is thinking about or what his mood is: sadness at losing an only daughter, concern for the cost of all the functions, etc., etc. The fact is that daddy at that moment was hoping he wouldn't fall during the trip down the aisle; he was in the midst of his long siege of stilt-leggedness and was walking on numbed feet and legs. Having had a year or more to practice walking on the afflicted limbs gave him some confidence, but falling in the midst of a wedding procession would somehow be different from falling anywhere else. The concern shows clearly in the picture. The paradox involved is that numbed legs and hypersensitivity of reflexes in the feet occurred simultaneously.

In this chapter a range of typical complaints or standard problems associated with multiple sclerosis have been explored. Awkward, inadvertent bumping into people, furniture and objects such as doorframes is one category of conventional problems. Lightheadedness and the correlated problem of nystagmus, aggression, and fatigue extended the list. Inability to focus attention for significant periods of time was explored as was the insidious nature of the earlier topic of fatigue. Hypersensitivity and numbness were again contrasted to remind you of the paradoxical nature of some pairs of symptoms.

To emphasize the reality of the symptoms, let me quote one of the self-help ideas in the *MS News*, Volume 2, Number 1. More will be said about this publication later. In the indicated issue contributor Marie Shapin says:

> For those of us who are numb in our hands and forearms and are not always aware that we have burned ourselves until the damage is done, bamboo tongs (available in any modern kitchenware section of a department store or through American Foundation for the Blind) are a must for extracting toast from the toaster.

One should remember that some of the more exotic symptoms such as layered vision, and numbness in but a single nerve, are widely known among MS patients. As suggested at the beginning of this chapter, a neurologist conversant with MS could accurately predict a half-dozen ailments suffered by any given patient. Yet particular symptoms can be so widely scattered that it is with some confidence neurologists say "every case is unique." Some of the symptoms are even suggestive of altogether different conditions or diseases, making early diagnosis a tricky assignment. These matters often weigh heavily on the patient and ill prepare him to learn that a physician, perhaps even a specialist, considers his case trivial, particularly when the diagnosis is not known by the patient.

One should bear in mind that a single symptom does not necessarily suggest that you have multiple sclerosis. Unless the new blood analysis technique, to be reported later, does indeed provide a single determinate test, physicians will continue to await and test patients for patterns of symptoms.

7
Characteristic Copings

Multiple sclerosis is not a killer. Somehow that is supposed to be a comforting thought. Perhaps it is comforting to know that you will continue to live even though you have been victimized by MS, but it is also distressing. Whether you endure type 2 MS, the immobilizing type 3, or some variant of either, the prospects seem grim. In such circumstances, any person reasonably normal in other respects must certainly attempt to rehearse for future possibilities, even while dealing with the everyday problems.

In short, you must cope. I am firmly convinced that to surrender is to worsen the condition. But what happens when the condition remains unknown? How then could one worsen his condition? Conversely, how could one cope with an unknown? To this point efforts have been made to indicate what happened to me during the dozen dim years as well as in the period after learning about my condition. It is a story of interest to me as I recall it. But this chapter is about "characteristic" ways of dealing with MS, and so the ideas and actions of many patients are offered for consideration.

Literature accompanying the annual appeal for funds by the Chicago Chapter of the National Multiple Sclerosis Society carries the following striking statement of belief by Dr. F.A. Davis, director of the Multiple Sclerosis Center at Rush-Presbyterian-St. Luke's Hospital in Chicago.

MS is not a killer. People with MS must learn to adapt to it and in order to do this they must understand it.

Something similar seems to have been on Susan L. Andrews' mind when at an American Psychological Association Symposium she said, "Multiple sclerosis is an affliction which demands an adjustive response from the afflicted." What are some of the adjustive responses characteristically found among MS patients?

One of my acquaintances says he has become more aggressive in many situations. Having progressed to the cane-using extension of type 2 he no longer can tolerate long waits for taxicabs. Neither can he endure standing during an entire train trip to his suburban home. "The little old ladies better stay out of my way," he says gesticulating as though warding off competitors for a cab with his cane and briefcase. He professes to the same combative spirit when seeking a seat on the train.

Other acquaintances with MS tell of becoming upset by faulty merchandise for which they paid full price, by the trick of advertising items which are not in stock, by persons getting ahead of them in a line, and so on through a lengthy list. The spouse of one of these complainers said to a group of us, "These seem like perfectly reasonable instances of appropriate indignation." Indeed, this may be a valid point. Nevertheless, many of us feel unable to restrain our sense of outrage in a variety of situations which others seem to ignore, and which we upon occasion have also dealt with in less obvious ways.

But MS patients who sometimes act in fits of near-mania also are subject to depression. In fact, one patient once suggested that the fatigue we all encounter may be but a manifestation of depression. Coping with depression is an individualized response. One says, "I paint," another, "I drive the car;" and others say they putter with flowers, cook, watch TV, read, or work. And nearly all agree that weeping, crying, even sobbing, is used to reduce or relieve feelings of depression.

A general characterization of many of the responses to depression is that they are disciplined responses. You perform your work as best you can in an orderly fashion, or you turn to tasks you have learned through self direction, tasks which have become habit for you but which you still enjoy. Such tasks are not necessarily frivolous or trivial. Some can be cyclical or seasonal chores which require hard work, but they all involve a disciplining routine which perhaps temporarily thwarts the engulfing mood of depression.

It has been said that once you realize you are in a depressed state, you are already beginning to feel better. Such is not necessarily the case for MS patients. Once realizing their state they must strive to combat it if only temporarily. Even a physically well person could develop severe psychological problems were he to overlay uncertainty and fear with depression. So attention to means for relieving depression is quite important for the MS patient.

You may recall the young mother mentioned earlier. She reported finding herself maneuvered by her mother-in-law into going shopping when it was but an idle pursuit, or attending a meeting merely as a companion for her in-law. This kind of situation is potentially explosive among persons who are well, but it is debilitating and therefore a source of many difficulties both physical and psychological for the MS patient. Ann knew that the response ". . . I just don't feel up to it" would be treated as an excuse for avoiding the invitation. Some of Ann's friends told her that she, and MS patients in general, did not have the option of delaying actions because of the judgments precipitated by such actions. If being a shopping companion uses the energy needed later to deal with the children, one must forthrightly decline invitations, avoid entrapments, and resist pressures to become a shopping companion, they said. Anyone who is skeptical about the impact of MS on the patient's energy or who challenges decisions based squarely on the fact that energy is lower is not entitled to consideration by the patient. These are hard, perhaps cruel words, but the patient's condition is real, and the underlying cause is merciless. To procrastinate about decisions of the kind being considered here is to lose ground in the struggle against MS. The apparent choice is an apparition; to be misled is folly.

The problem with an in-law brings to mind the general question of deciding whom to inform about your condition. There are other in-law stories to recount, but we will decline the temptation in favor of addressing a very knotty problem area: When, how, and for what reasons does the family inform others of the patient's condition?

This area of questions is pressing particularly, perhaps exclusively, for the patient with type 2 MS, or extensions thereof, but who is ambulatory. Perhaps obviously, the type 3 patient, dependent upon a wheelchair, or the bedfast patient of type 4 could hide their condition only through complicated ruses; and none to my knowledge has attempted to hide his condition in such fashion. But type 2 MS patients have voiced concern over whether or not to tell the boss. Some have experienced indecision about informing friends, particularly those with whom they share an athletically oriented activity. Bowling, tennis, golfing, some kinds of fishing, all suffer either because of the reduction of coordination of the MS patient, or because of the extra demand made on the patient's energy. Should you try to plug along participating or simply be honest, both with yourself and friends?

Friends provide part of the clue to one good answer. This answer has been used as the basis for a decision by many MS patients. One part of the reasoning is that friends are accepting one of another. Thus distress over revealing that you suffer from this relatively unknown disease is reduced. Friends won't think you any different than before they knew of your disease. Somehow friends sort out the person from the ailment, treating you as a personality and the ailment as an accident. Further, they are quite willing to share your burden best they can, either by listening, discussing, or doing nothing, whichever seems your preference.

Acquaintances, on the other hand, are less likely to be prepared to empathize. Not knowing you as well as friends, acquaintances are more likely to confuse accident and person, being less able to identify the person apart from the accident. Consequently any tale of woe from you is unlikely to do more than irritate them. Complete disinterest, following a few seconds of attention, is the most likely possibility. In fact, even friends will act more like acquaintances if over-exposed to a recounting of the trials and tribulations of either the patient or the spouse. Constant association of complaints and personality no doubt leads friends to act more like acquaintances, confusing you and the accident of your condition. As in other matters, the boundary line of over-exposure is drawn at unpredictably different places by everyone.

The decision we made about whom to inform follows a guideline drawn from the suggestions of fellow patients and spouses. It can be stated as follows: persons who have a right or need to know, because their interactions with you will be altered necessarily, should be informed in a manner reflecting the stating of a matter of fact which has consequences.

In our case the implementation of this rule-of-thumb was perhaps somewhat easier because some of my limitations had already become apparent before I was informed of the diagnosis. We learned this when we informed our minister and heard him say, among other things of a more religious nature, "This puts a lot of things in context, it provides pieces for a number of puzzles." Recalling his musings I could easily imagine some of the incomplete puzzles with which my actions had burdened him. One no doubt was: "I wonder why he left the dinner table twice during our dinner with the editorial director of the Daily News?" Another probably was: "I wonder why he abandoned his leadership roles in the church?" The first, of course, was connected to the hypersensitivity syndrome which worked on the bladder sensors. The second was directly related to the problem of fatigue which was at one of its periodic peaks at the time we advised him of the nature of my condition.

Another person whom we admitted to the small circle who knew of my condition was my boss. As chairman of the department his responsibilities embraced the appointment of committees, recommendations for increases in salary and promotions in rank, and overseeing developments which would provide budget-savings as well as enhance the reputation of the institution. At the beginning of his second year in office I told him of the MS problem. Kay and I were following the "right-to-know" rule, but I found myself offering two reasons for the timing of the disclosure. First, having held office for a full year, the chairman had had opportunity to make at least tentative plans for the department, and, thus, opportunity to decide what, if any, role I was to play. Second, it was about this time that I began to accept the diagnosis fully enough to talk about it, even haltingly.

One acquaintance did not inform his boss until the time when a promotion was offered. At that point the acquaintance felt that to accept the promotion without disclosing his condition would have been to run the risk of perpetrating a fraud. Not only was the promotion made, but subsequently he was promoted a second time. Later his condition worsened somewhat, but he reported no move to replace him or to shift him to a less productive position. Neither did he seem to think he was unable to do the work.

Another episode taught us something more about disclosing the MS condition to friends. We were attending a gala weekend celebration of one couple's thirtieth wedding anniversary. The dozen or so people attending were among the honorees' best friends so there was no lack of common interests in golf, dancing, bridge, and informal chatting. One of the men suffered from Parkinson's disease, and so was among the less active, resting fairly regularly throughout the period. However, he was far from being excluded, and was treated as naturally in the group as though he were free of any ailment. Over the years he had simply carved a new role with the help of the group, and no disruption of the group was visible or discernible.

We have not yet disclosed my MS to the couple whose party we attended. Situations which might present an appropriate occasion for disclosure have not yet arisen. The situation most likely to precipitate the announcement to this couple is a game of golf. I have always been a duffer, and it is no surprise to them that even duffers have relatively bad days on the links. Furthermore, my friend became addicted to the golf cart early enough so that my use of a cart to ward off fatigue did not arouse suspicion. They have a right to know, and we will tell them when the condition affects our interactions. As of now the appropriate situation has not arisen.

There is yet another consideration which weighs on the decision to inform others of your condition. This consideration is a personal one. It stems from a need to have your burden shared. Kay tells me that during the long years of her secret suffering, she became unable to keep the information private. She took a friend of long standing into her confidence. This friend, predictably, shared the burden, kept the secret, at least from me, and apparently thought no less of either of us. Kay has reciprocated, sharing the friend's troubles in similar manner.

Other types of coping are less complex than wrestling with the problem of announcing that you have MS. Some of these types of coping are directly related to one or another symptoms. For example, the weakness and numbness of the legs is difficult to ignore. One acquaintance with MS is always in a hurry. Also, he is a person who brought to his condition a history of always thinking it better to do things himself than to rely on others. Thus, rather than bother his family to bring him a towel or a book, he prefers to fetch such things himself; besides he thinks he can do it faster. He often falls at home because his legs are not in good enough shape, either sensorily or strengthwise, to accommodate his dispositions. Ever so slowly he is learning to slow down and to permit others to do chores for him. Fortunately he seems able to assess himself in a relatively objective manner, noting the humor in pratfalls stemming from his own foolishness. My own problems with regard to legs, you may recall, were somewhat less severe, leading primarily to bumps, bruises, and slightly damaged furniture. But such experiences tend to slow one down and to cause one to rethink the do-it-yourself attitude.

Another common symptom which requires coping is

loss of memory. This loss is two-fold. First, there is a loss of memory for words, in my case primarily nouns. Second, there is loss of memory for tasks. What was I supposed to do? Let me hasten to add that the loss, in the case of words, is not really a loss of memory. Rather, it seems to me to be a failure of the retrieval system of the mind. My evidence is to be found in the action I learned to take when "memory failed."

Eight or ten years before my physician informed me of the diagnosis, it became apparent to me that an occasional word failed to appear as needed in my speech. The lapse first came to my attention while teaching. My characteristic role as teacher in the classroom includes both lecturing and discussion with students. Both of these oral roles offer opportunity for the type of memory failure involving single words. At first it seemed possible to find a substitute word after but a flicker of a pause. (The fact that this happened would seem to provide evidence that my thoughts are in the form of meanings rather than words. How else could an alternate word be selected for a word which I had apparently forgotten?) This coping by substitution soon led me to realize that the original word sought had not been forgotten. Shortly after the hesitation and substitution, the original word sought would occur to me. Apparently an unconscious search through alternate routes was set off at the pause-and-substitute point. This led me to test the proposition that an unconscious search for lost words was more successful than a conscious one. From time to time I directed all conscious efforts to the retrieval of a lost word. Never did this succeed in retrieval in as short a period as did the unconscious search, apparently undertaken when you plunge on with a substitute, not stopping to show concern over your faulty memory.

An acquaintance, recently struck by a type 3 condition, was having difficulty recalling a word for a sentence from time to time during conversations. Once a successful engineer, he was now mobile only by wheelchair, and had not yet accepted the fact that he had MS. When in the course of a conversation he forgot a word, he would persevere in attempts to recall that word, sometimes clenching a fist, sometimes bowing his head, sometimes striking the table vigorously with his hand. Others of us who had learned to cope with this situation urged him to forego his persistence and try alternative coping behaviors. He was not yet ready to submit to the notion that slight loss of memory was a fact of life for many MS patients; he persisted in attempting to overcome the symptom through willpower.

Returning to the second type of loss of memory, forgetting tasks, let me assure you that it is sometimes amusing. I was urged to write out a schedule of activities and responsibilities each morning when I reached the office. So far as I know, I never failed to arrive at work, but sometimes I have forgotten to make a list. One day, several years ago, I answered the telephone and found myself talking to a man about twenty or twenty-five miles away. He asked if I weren't supposed to be in his office at that moment attending a meeting prior to carrying out other activities in his school in the afternoon. The answer was "Yes." A car rental had to be arranged before starting to the meeting already in progress but the details of that can be skipped over. The activities for the afternoon were undertaken more or less successfully.

My good wife has learned to come to my rescue at times when there is a great deal to think about, or a long list to remember. She has taken to making out a list for me before we leave home. In turn, I have learned to put the list in a conspicuous place so as not to forget I have it. The top-left handkerchief pocket of my suit coat or jacket is a good spot. But folding the list so it protrudes from the pocket has been a useful extra precaution. This type of loss of memory seems to be quite different from the loss of an occasional word. Spontaneous recovery of the information sought is not characteristic of this second kind of forgetting.

Hypersensitivity has been mentioned. It seems to be a typical symptom and one which it is impossible to ignore. At a meeting of couples, one member of each of whom was afflicted by MS, one of the women said, "Let's face it. We are all hypersensitive." She was not referring to psychological sensitivity. Rather, she meant literal physical hypersensitivity, some kind of irritation of the nerves themselves.

In my case, hypersensitivity manifested itself in several ways. I have already cited the example of the itching ear and scalp, and the episode of "stilt legs" which now is seen as a paradox, for accompanying the numbness of the stilt legs was the maddening symptom of hypersensitivity.

The hypersensitivity half of the paradox floats into action on occasion even today. I can recall vividly having this condition in 1965, for Kay and I took a few days off to enjoy the mineral baths, massages, and horse races in Hot Springs, Arkansas. As I learned two or three years ago, this was an unfortunate decision regarding the hot baths, for an increase in body temperature exacerbates many of the problems symptomatic of MS.

One of the recurring symptoms involves the legs. It is knee-jerking, a very common complaint among the MS patients known to me. Occurring primarily at night, it can rob you of sleep. The other recurring symptom is having sensitive feet. One might say the feet are extremely ticklish. This symptom is not confined to the bedtime hours. It can haunt you in the middle of an interview, while teaching, during a bus ride, or any time, it seems. When this symptom is operative I always warn the physician that he is in danger of being kicked during the testing of reflexes in the feet. My right foot seems more severely affected than does the left. However, both are capable of distracting my attention from tasks at hand.

Although the exact time of onset of this hypersensitivity escapes me, when it occurred it caused me to reevaluate my ideas about my condition. Having suffered numbness in the right hand, right leg and buttock, and across the belly, I had become accustomed to thinking in terms of numbness. The realization that hypersensitivity had set in led me to tell my physician that I would have to begin using the phrase "altered sensation" to cover the two manifestations. Some of my time was spent subsequently in attempts to sort the altered sensations more carefully into the categories "numb" and "hypersensitive," a differentiation which was a little difficult to accomplish at first.

Hypersensitivity of the feet is a condition which apparently can be precipitated by ingredients in several widely used beverages such as coffee, colas, and cocoa. This, as you might guess, is information which was not offered to me for a dozen or more years. Not knowing what the condition was nor what to do about symptoms, I developed an inappropriate idea about how to cope. Having read a little about nerves and synapses in psychology books over the years, I knew that once a nerve "fired," that is, an impulse was passed along, that there was a tiny interval of time required before it could fire again. Somehow I arrived at the idea that perhaps the firing mechanism could be worn out as a person becomes fatigued and made inoperative for an undefined but long interval. If so, some relief from the hypersensitive condition might be obtained. I undertook the chore of rubbing my feet with a firm application of the fingertips so that the various reflexes around the edges of the feet and across the bottom would be activated over and over again. But very little relief was developed from this exercise; independent jerking resumed almost immediately. Nevertheless, the actions were continued almost as though

I were driven to the task. One of the objects which make the 1965 Hot Springs trip so vivid in memory is the rough fiber mitt with which the attendant rubs your body, legs, and feet during the hot bath. I still have my first such mitt on the soap shelf of one of our bathrooms. It was used a good many times to rub my feet while bathing in the vain hope of gaining some relief from the hypersensitive reflexes.

In time I discovered that untrimmed toenails seemed to be accompanied by a minimal return of the hypersensitive foot problem. And, indeed, a careful trimming and shaping of the nails does seem to alleviate the condition when it is not severe.

From conversations with other MS patients it seems clear that drugs of one kind or another can now be used to alleviate the hypersensitivity syndrome. If so, I rejoice for all those who in this way can escape the insistent demands this symptom makes on both energy and attention. If this symptom recurs too often I anticipate requesting a relief-giving drug.

Several objects serve as symbols of types of MS. The cane, the walker, the wheelchair, and the bed all symbolize degrees of affliction. These, then, become symbols which must be rejected by the patient. The general degree of severity of many MS patients I know is type 2 bordering on type 3. To them the cane is recommended as a steadying factor in walking. At this point patients appear to have an identical reaction. They say, "Well, I'll just buy a cheap cane because I won't be needing it very long," and they do just that. Before many weeks have passed they purchase a sturdy, substantial cane, for they realize it is to be their companion for a very long time. Even then, not all patients can accept the cane. One fellow, at this stage of the disease, purchased a cane with a screw-on handle and a hollow top. The top holds four one- or two-ounce vials which enable him to mix his favorite cocktail upon request. Of course, this feature is also a conversation piece which enables everyone to acknowledge the cane without accepting or mentioning the patient's physical condition.

Another method of coping with MS is characteristic of more men than women, primarily because more men presently are responsible for the feeding, sheltering, and clothing of a family. This coping takes the form of arranging affairs in anticipation of becoming disabled. In my case, disclosure of the condition was withheld for many years. When finally informed, I deemed it necessary to move with all possible speed in arranging and understanding the financial situation we would face were I to become disabled. You see, learning that MS is a progressive, degenerative disease puts you in a state of urgency. Discovering that it has been working on you for at least twelve years raises urgency to near-panic.

There were surprises awaiting me, some pleasant, some aggravating. Among the more pleasant surprises was my employer's attitude toward retirement for an employee. I learned that a disabled employee would have full payments made into his retirement fund until age 65. This means that at age 65 the disabled employee would have a handsome retirement plan only slightly affected by disability. The slight reduction in the retirement fund would result because the employee presumably would not benefit from salary increases after the time of establishment of disability.

Another pleasant surprise was the realization that Social Security would pay the disabled worker monthly an amount equal to his benefits at normal retirement age. These payments, if applied for, would start three months after the established date of disability.

One of the disappointing surprises was learning that the long-term disability group plan in which my colleagues and I enrolled was inferior to another well-known plan. I was not searching extensively for the best plan available, merely comparing our plan with the plan offered by the organization which already handled our retirement plan. My rough calculations suggested that the plan in which we were enrolled would pay approximately $100 per month less than the plan offered by the organization which we entrust with our regular retirement funds.

But this disappointment was to be followed by repeated aggravation because no one in the administrative hierarchy would entertain seriously the possibility of reconsidering the matter of compensation during disability.

I first took the matter to my departmental chairman. Perhaps it is important to say that at no time during the series of events reported here did anyone in the university with whom I raised the matter of benefits know that I suffered from multiple sclerosis. Lacking this knowledge they might have considered my inquiry to be merely irritating meddling in a matter of little consequence.

When the matter was raised with the chairman, he suggested that it be referred to one of our representatives on the Council of the Senate, the ruling body of the faculty. One of my councilmen received my inquiry and informed me, following the next meeting of the council, of a message from a fellow member of the council, a man from the law school. The message was that the administration had asked for a new bid on an improved disability plan, and information about the matter should be forthcoming. There ensued a period of silent waiting that lasted a year. During this period we elected a new departmental chairman.

A year is a long time to await word about your disability benefits when, so far as you know, the next attack of your disease might be the one to disable you. I made inquiry again to the councilman. He said he had heard nothing further about the matter. When I asked if he would inquire he said, "This is not really the business of the senate or its council. We deal with academic matters and you are asking about an administrative matter." When I reminded the councilman that our departmental chairman directed my inquiry to him, he said that the chairman had been wrong in so doing. He did not say anything about the fact that he had reported having made inquiry after my first contact. At this time the relative insignificance of the matter to the previous chairman and to the councilman occurred to me.

The matter could not be left as it was, for I was still very concerned to ensure as high disability payments as possible. I wrote to the new chairman, stating the history of the inquiry and asking his advice. He recommended that I contact the comptroller. I did, and talked with the man in charge of the disability plan. He sounded somewhat disinterested and double-talked and said, "Well, there are so many different plans that it is hard to keep track." It was evident to me that he felt an individual had no business disturbing anyone about a group matter. Clearly there were channels of communication and authority to be followed. Unfortunately I had attempted to use these channels, and was rebuked. I decided that the aggravation was detrimental and more difficult to endure than would be the lower disability funds. Pursuit of this inquiry was terminated, but not without some sorrow. Within a community of thoughtful, sensitive people it was possible for a distressed individual to be thwarted repeatedly while pursuing a matter of primary importance to him and of interest, if not immediate concern, to the entire community.

Coping, then, at times includes the rearrangement of priorities among concerns, particularly when you discover that there is no way to satisfy, relieve or cure the focus of concern. Reducing your zest for immediate action rather than falling, taking little notice of the partial loss of memory rather than trying to will your memory into action, accepting the prospect of a lesser retirement income rather than attempting to arouse essentially disinterested colleagues—all these seem to be examples of the rearrangement of priorities.

I would not want to end consideration of coping on such a fundamentally sorrowful note. There are many things which type 2 and type 3 MS patients do which are more positive than rearranging priorities, important as the latter is. One such positive coping is to exercise. Unused muscles can atrophy, and where messages fail to be transmitted in the nervous system there are likely to be unused muscles. Nearly every MS patient I have known has a pattern of exercises done daily. These stimulate circulation, and keep muscles toned up so they will remain strong enough to be used, even if only for limited activity.

In my case the exercising seemed to be something which I felt ought to be done, even though I was ignorant of the need for exercise for my undisclosed disease. Fortunately my interest became focused on a book which provided detailed directions for a large number of exercises done by those interested in yoga. My interest was only in exercising, and I found the eight, ten, or twelve exercises to be useful, fun, and interesting. Muscles which had remained unknown to me suddenly came to my attention. I realized how puny and halfhearted all the physical education and calisthenics programs of my schooling and army life had been. Through time and because of inattention my ability to perform all the exercises accomplished at first has diminished. However, a few of the original exercises plus an occasional new addition for a specific purpose have been part of my daily regimen for a decade or more.

Perhaps I shall never cease to wonder what lead me to these exercises, but I shall always be grateful that the exercises were undertaken. There is not question in my mind about the part they played in my life. The requirement of equal dexterity with right and left limbs and the necessity for controlled balance in the exercises required daily practice which undoubtedly helped me manage a tortuous path through the lengthy stilt-legs episode without the necessity for a cane. Similarly, perhaps even more directly, the eye exercises and various head-down positions enabled me to accommodate more readily the lightheadedness and dizziness which, characteristically of MS, occurred from time to time.

Exercising, as has been said, is one of the copings with positive outcomes. Another category is eating habits. One fact which comes to you with the speed of gossip once you have made contact with a group of MS patients, is that caffein leads to the irritation of nerves. Some neurologists believe that the heat of the beverage, rather than the caffein, is responsible for the irritability in MS patients. My own history attests to the possibility that the elimination of caffein from the diet of an MS patient has a dramatic effect.

Dr. Davis speaks the truth when he says that MS requires adaptation which in turn requires understanding of the condition. It is possible that for years I could have accommodated and adapted to the condition had I know its identity. I am thankful that one way or another some methods of coping occurred naturally to me.

8

Current Considerations

Perhaps the reader can excuse the extensive use of first person in this book. This is really not meant to be simply my story, but you must understand that MS is a personal disease. My hope is to have conveyed some of the difficulties, stresses, and trauma of the MS patient, even the one so fortunate as to have avoided the wheelchair and the bed. The permutations and combinations of symptoms which an ingenious condition of MS can generate are startling. My own symptoms and episodes are well known to me, and therefore enable this attempt to convey feelings and thoughts which I could not successfully elicit from others; feelings and thoughts which, nevertheless, are like those of other patients.

Type 2 MS, thinking in terms of the four type description of Chapter II is far from the worst condition which might strike one. But it renders you in far from the best physical or mental condition as you can imagine. Strange, persisting numbness catches your attention from time to time. Odd hints at lightheadedness and vertigo cross your consciousness at unpredictable moments. In spite of an ordinarily effective drug program, a sphincter valve, or its controlling sensor may revert to a balky stage. Dependent perhaps on your general physical condition, one or both legs may jerk at night, disturbing your otherwise peaceful rest. And double, or rather layered, vision seems to lurk about, perhaps as a friendly indicator of overwork by the eyes. For those with an extended type 2 diagnosis there is the hovering specter of a wheelchair awaiting an opportunity to replace the cane.

I am mindful of the symptoms in store should my type 2 blossom into type 3 or even type 4. And I am thankful for having been spared a worse condition. But in a way sufferers of type 2 are doubly jeopardized. They are stricken with a number of symptoms which have been discussed in this book. They are likely to suffer partial loss of word memory, to become fatigued easily, and to stumble as they walk. But they are in double jeopardy, knowing not but what the next attack will render them immobile, perhaps completely dependent on others. It has been said that man spends his life anxiously avoiding trauma; that when you have been traumatized, life becomes somewhat easier because you have lost your anxiety. Perhaps so, but there are many MS patients who feel that they have been traumatized by type 2 or 3 MS, and yet must anxiously anticipate the possibility that they might be more severely stricken at any time. That seems like double jeopardy to me.

In fact, a case might be made for triple jeopardy for patients with type 2 MS. It should be apparent that patients who seem to lack obvious physical impairment are always suspect if they beg off any activity; in their own eyes as well as in the eyes of others such patients seem to be "using" MS as an excuse. Furthermore, the occasional patient who endures attack after attack without knowledge of what is transpiring has the haunting thought that his problems are psychosomatic. These kinds of psychic trauma seem to impose the third phase of triple jeopardy.

We have dealt briefly with methods of coping with MS. In the more severe types it has been my observation that the patient must come to realize that others are willing to help. Such help should be viewed as freely given by one human to another. The patient and his helpmate are but part of a grand web of humanity. Somehow, sometime the patient or a third human will help yet another, and in such fashion repayment to the first helpmate is made in full. It appears to be easy to stir up evil with its seemingly endless repercussions, and very difficult to either arouse good or to see its effects beyond the immediate case. But perhaps we've got it all wrong. Perhaps in its own quiet, imperceptible way the kind word or the silent deed has manifold consequences yet unknown.

Whether it be ego protection or simply habit which tends to prevent the patient from accepting offers of assistance, even type 2 MS patients must learn to surmount the barrier and accept freely such offers. Part of the difficulty which patients have in dealing with assistance offered is that they have not as yet accepted the fact that they are ill, that they do suffer some degree of affliction corresponding to one or another well-defined type of MS.

If you are fortunate enough to have avoided being afflicted by one of the "dread" diseases, perhaps talk about not yet accepting the fact that you have such a disease is puzzling, even unintelligible to you. But it is believable to many who have been so stricken. At first, not only are you unable to talk about it, you may not be able to hold the idea in conscious memory long enough to think about it. When the fact is thus buried, you have no reason to believe or accept it. You may deal with it objectively, but be unable to even think about it in relationship to yourself. In my own case, I read extensively about MS as soon as the physician revealed my diagnosis. Yet over two years later I was barely able to utter the words, "I have multiple sclerosis" to my wife. Another year elapsed before I was able to disclose this information to a second person whom we thought ought to know. Yet another half year sped past before I was able to discuss the condition with my daughter, in spite of the fact that I knew she was well prepared by training, education, and past information to discuss it.

This personal experience leads me to say that MS patients should try to accept offers of assistance even if they must be thought of in terms of courtesy rather than in terms of help. If you must wait until you can think and talk about your situation before you are prepared to accept assistance, you may be in for a long wait, and others may be mistakenly led to believe that you are stubborn, or ungrateful.

Once you begin to make progress in accepting your affliction, a variety of methods of coping can open before you. Some patients exercise to keep key muscles toned up, thus hoping to prevent atrophy in a muscle which temporarily may be used very little. Some, as we have seen, delight in their new role as aggressor in the struggle for seating on public transportation, or in hailing and landing a taxi.

Some, and here our remarks extend to persons with a wide range of types of MS, become involved in the "home-bound" program for MS patients. This program, using trained personnel and special vehicles capable of accommodating patients in wheelchairs, offers an unbelievable array of activities: bowling, swimming, sewing, camping, grooming, shopping, and crafts being among those offered by the Chicago Chapter of the National Multiple Sclerosis Society.

In Chicago there are also two MS centers. My contact has been with the one at the Rush-Presbyterian-St. Luke's

Medical Center. This MS center has been active in research, not only on the physical condition known as MS but also on the psychological implications of the disease. One of the programs of this center has been described by Marcia Pavlou, Ph.D., program coordinator for the center, in the papers from the American Psychological Association symposium. (The symposium referred to throughout most of the remainder of this chapter is the one referenced in the preface.)

The Program of Comprehensive Health Care for the Multiple Sclerosis Patient is primarily a short-term program for outpatients. With spouses they are invited to attend discussion groups which are "directed primarily toward the psychiatrically normal individual undergoing unusual long-term stress." Each group meets perhaps twice a month for a half-dozen or so discussions, although some groups continue longer, and some couples continue from year to year by joining other groups. Two psychologists led the first group to which Kay and I belonged. Dr. Davis, neurologist and director of the center, spoke at one meeting, and consults with the psychologists. His presentation included a description of various types of MS and some conceptualization of its basic nature. The four types of MS referred to in this book were presented by Dr. Davis. For most spouses, and some patients, this was the first time they had been given this kind of information. Several remarked how interesting and useful his very short presentation on MS had been.

We continued to have telephone contact for a year with one other patient from the first group, and we are always interested in hearing about other members of the group. We are now in our third group. From time to time I see one or another member of one of the groups during my Tuesday afternoon visits to the center.

The purposes for the discussion groups provide some insight into the problems MS patients face. Dr. Pavlou stated four purposes:

1. From an informational frame of reference, relate the medical management of the disease to the patient's understanding of his disease, its implications, and his expectations.
2. Provide a structured opportunity for patients to deal with their own experiences and reactions as MS patients, identify and facilitate adaptive changes in lifestyles, goals, and expectations.
3. Provide a supportive environment where more sensitive issues can be discussed with others undergoing similar stress. These include physical control and mobility, problems of bowel and bladder function, problems of sexual function and adaption.
4. Provide an opportunity for patients to explore family reactions to MS in terms of impact on family life, vocational planning, and interpersonal functioninig.

Kay and I have found the discussion groups to be of inestimable value. As a direct result of participation in our first group, and with her urging, I began to accept my MS sufficiently to be able to inform my employer of my condition. We also began to share discussions with our grown daughter, and the three of us plan to attempt to attend the annual luncheon meeting of the Chicago Chapter of the National Multiple Sclerosis Society. One year I attended alone, and one year my daughter and I managed to attend.

Those in attendance at the first annual luncheon I attended included an interesting range of persons involved with MS. Most, of course, were patients, but one man at our table was there seeking any information or sign of hope which he might carry home to his invalid daughter. On my left sat a mid-twentyish lady who had been helped dramatically by ACTH. Bedridden for several years, she was now mobile with but slight symptoms of ataxia. Here certainly was more than a ray of hope for the man across from us. But no. His daughter had already put ACTH to the test, with no apparent effect on the course of the MS. It seemed as though they had tried everything known with no effect. And so it goes. Each case seems unique, with some having unsettling consequences. As Dr. William Cammin stated in his paper at the APA symposium, "The profound post-diagnosis impact upon the adjustment of both the individual patient and the family of the MS patient would be eased if the MS patient could avail himself of psychological techniques."

Lest you forget my suggestion of a continuous battle against the idea that my problems were psychosomatic, read another point made by Dr. Cammin: "The early diagnosis of MS is frequently difficult and many times results in the patient being referred to a psychiatrist or clinical psychologist for treatment." This has the unfortunate effect of validating the physician's diagnosis, for as Dr. Cammin says, "Many times a mental health professional who treats the MS patient is unfamiliar with MS and proceeds to treat the individual as though the primary problem is mental." Please bear in mind that the symposium was held in 1974, not 1964 or 1874.

The range of persons attending the annual luncheons suggests that it is not only the MS patient who is deeply concerned. Dr. Cammin's statements reinforce the belief that families also are victimized by MS. The sum of patients plus their immediate families suggests that a rather large number of persons are directly concerned with MS. In order that you might draw your own inference about how many people in this country are involved with MS, let me provide some information.

The number of persons in the United States who suffer

affliction by multiple sclerosis may be much higher than the official estimate. The definition of affliction can vary from one neurologist to the next. Even the very useful definitions of types of MS found herein have fuzzy boundaries which are not helpful in establishing firm figures on the total number of MS patients in the country. Recent annual figures from the National Institute of Neurological Diseases and Blindness show an estimated half-million persons in the United States afflicted with multiple sclerosis and other closely related neurological disorders. That would be an estimate of one out of every 400 or 500 persons in the country. Add one or two concerned persons for every patient and you could have one out of every 100 or 200 involved closely with multiple sclerosis.

There is a long list of additional topics related to MS which one might explore. For example, there has been little or no hint of mortality figures for MS patients. Nor has the topic of divorce been broached, nor suicide. All three topics confront you if you read technical sociological literature on MS patients, or mingle with those afflicted. A variety of reasons might be offered to rationalize lack of attention to these and other topics, but the fundamental reason is that there is a paucity of information available. It seems that few investigators have found such topics as interesting as problems related to the disease itself. Consequently, topics such as geographic distribution of MS, topography of the patches of scars on the central neural system, and fundamental cause of the disease receive attention while topics such as mortality rate, and others mentioned above tend to be ignored. But the attraction of problems more centrally focused on the disease does not entirely explain the paucity of information about other topics. Consideration of mortality figures may help you understand this assertion.

Several national studies of mortality among MS patients have been completed. Many of them are reported in *Acta Neurologica Scandinavia.* For example, studies from Finland (1975) and the Netherlands (1973) are to be found there. Some data for the United States, Denmark, and Norway are in the 1972 volume of the same journal. Leibowitz and Alter published a book *Multiple Sclerosis, Clues to Its Cause* in 1973; it was a study done in Israel. A common problem for all the authors was to determine the date of onset of the disease. If they used a category like "longevity after onset of MS" they had to define "onset" as "diagnosis" although in many if not most cases the date of onset is obviously months or years before the diagnosis. The same diffculty arose when the investigators attempted to divide patients into two categories of "Age at onset of MS."

Various attempts to ascribe death to MS have encountered another problem as vexing as determining onset of the disease. We have seen that MS can affect any function dependent in part on activity of the central neural system. This has led (or driven) investigators to report deaths among MS patients categorized by initial presenting symptom. One such list of categories included motor, sensory, visual, diplopia, cerebellar-vestibular, and sphincter among a total of nine. Clearly more deaths are traceable to multiple sclerosis than the phrase "not a killer" might suggest. When I began investigating this topic it was aggravating to find no mortality figures for MS. The longer I looked the more I realized the problems which investigators faced. However, some figures on life span of MS patients regardless of cause of death might be interesting.

In view of the fact that the 1974 symposium reflects information about MS as fresh as any available to the general public, perhaps it would be interesting to examine the papers more closely. It appears that we have already found them useful in discussions of MS, so let's take a more intensive look.

In the preface we have already identified the persons who prepared papers for the symposium. The symposium, to refresh your memory, was entitled "Psychology and Health: Clinical Psychological Services to Multiple Sclerosis Patients." Michael F. Hartings, Ph.D., organized and chaired the symposium at the annual meeting of the American Psychological Association which was held in New Orleans in 1974. All the papers for this symposium were prepared and read by psychologists except the one by Floyd A. Davis, M.D., who has previously been identifed as director of the Rush Multiple Sclerosis Center in Chicago. You are reminded that references to Dr. Schwartz' words come from his contribution to the Symposium Proposal, for I have not seen the paper he was scheduled to present.

It is interesting to note casually the topics addressed by the authors, and the relative emphasis given to each. Psychological problems associated with MS were addressed by all five authors. Adaptive needs, although singled out for discussion by only two of the five authors, received the second heaviest emphasis. Discussions of personality factors, as either contributing to or resulting from MS, were included by two authors, and emphasized by only one. Impairment of brain function was mentioned by two, although examined by only one of these two authors. Only the neurologist spoke of MS in clinical terms although one other author alluded to symptoms of the disease.

The psychological problems these investigators reported were drawn primarily from direct observation of MS patients in discussion groups, and from the research literature in one paper. Davis said, "The disease is therefore a crippler and not a killer and presents a most trying situation both for the professionals involved in clinical management and, of course, the patient, who must learn somehow to adapt to this devastating disease."

Even the title of Andrews' paper suggested problems: "Cognitive, Emotional and Personality Correlates of Multiple Sclerosis." She reported that "depression and euphoria are effects typically attributed to organic pathology." Our earlier references to fatigue and depression, and the comments made by members of a discussion group are reflected in one of the conclusions from research reported by Andrews: "The depression seen in persons with MS is best regarded as reactive, psychogenic depression and not a function of Central Nervous System damage." In the same vein as Davis, Andrews thinks of MS as involving "a crisis of adjustment." Touching on some of our earlier concerns, she said, "The person's symptoms may prohibit him from continuing to live a full and normal life, but at the same time are not severe enough for him to receive social approval for adopting the role of invalid."

In her paper describing the discussion group aspect of comprehensive care at Rush, Pavlou made the startling statement that: "The group meets a second need, that of providing support during a time similar to that experienced during the mourning process." The loss, in the case of MS, is "loss of functioning and . . . loss of identity as a healthy individual." The group also permits the patient to realize that this depression, anger, fear and confusion are not new states among MS patients, according to Pavlou.

According to Cammin, among the major factors influencing psychological adjustment in cases of MS is the patient's state of emotional adjustment prior to being stricken. Even the well-adjusted person will probably "react with anger, frustration, and depression at the very real and traumatic limitations inherent in the diagnosis." But "he will accept these more readily and adjust his life style accordingly, more quickly" than others less well-adjusted before the occurrence of MS.

It would be difficult to deny that patients with MS

suffer psychological problems in view of the unanimous opinion of the symposium participants, who offered evidence from both direct observation and research reports. Throughout this book an attempt has been made to convey the nature of some of these problems through personal episodes as well as by reports from and about others.

One of the areas of concern which has been ignored by your author, up to this point, is damage to brain function. Davis suggests that "organic mental syndromes . . . do not form a substantial part of the clinical picture." However, "non-organic mental dysfunction is usually rampant."

Andrews, in summarizing research since about 1950, stated two generalizations:

1. Whenever subjects with multiple sclerosis have been compared with non-brain-damaged subjects on measures reflecting intellectual efficiency, the performance of the subjects with MS has either been significantly poorer, or poorer but not significantly so. Not one comparison in the data which I have reviewed has shown MS subjects to score higher than non-brain-damaged subjects. . . .
2. Whenever subjects with multiple sclerosis have been compared with subjects having other organic brain damage, the performance of the two groups has been quite similar.

Andrews reported a study of MS patients by Surridge who "found intellectual impairment to be distributed as follows: none—39%, slight—41%, moderate—14% and severe—6%." She is attempting to construct a case for believing "that MS often results in an organically induced impairment of intellectual efficiency."

Of interest in connection with discussions of possible brain damage resulting from MS is a news report filed by Donald McLachlan. At one point in the report he said that

Professor Ephraim Field, lecturer in experimental pathology at England's University of Newcastle, "explained that because of the low levels of linoleic acid in MS victims, white blood cells become rampant and attack the brain." A direct quotation attributed to Professor Field states: "We conducted tests to measure the sensitivity of those cells in MS patients. And we found the reaction of the cells on the brain was reduced by 90 per cent by the use of linoleic acid." This evidence would support the contention that organic brain impairment is possible in MS. The point being made by Professor Field is that for the first time "through a blood sample test, we have a means of early detection for multiple sclerosis."

This, of course, would be of great importance, since MS is so difficult to diagnose early. Of great importance to diagnosed patients is a second item in McLachlan's report. Again the substance of interest is linoleic acid. This time the physician being quoted is Dr. Harold Millar, consultant neurologist at the Royal Victoria Hospital in Belfast, Northern Ireland. He too asserts that multiple sclerosis patients have a lowered amount of linoleic acid in their blood. Dr. Millar and his associates have successfully increased the quantity of linoleic acid in the blood by having patients drink a natural fluid containing a large amount of the acid. McLachlan reported that, "Dr. Millar said there were 62 relapses suffered over the two years among the 39 patients who did not receive (the) . . . oil. But he said there were only 41 relapses in the 36-member group that had been given the oil treatment." It was further pointed out by Dr. Millar that, "relapses—such as temporary loss of vision or weakness in the legs—were twice as severe in the untreated group as in the treated groups and of a longer duration."

Of course there have been hopeful signs before, ideas which led to nothing positive for patients although they may have cleared away some brush for future investigators. But the linoleic acid line is thought to have some substantial base in theory and thus stands a better chance of leading to outcomes both useful to research and helpful to patients.

Returning to the papers from the symposium, we have already noted the authors' discussion of psychological problems and brain damage, presumably related to and perhaps even caused by MS. The topic given the second heaviest emphasis was adaptive needs. We have already considered Ms. Pavlou's statement of the purposes for discussion groups at the Rush MS Center. Of the group experience she said it "is directed toward meeting a number of adaptive needs." Some of these needs, she suggested, are: information "about the nature and course of the disease, research, and available treatments." She pointed out that information needs to be repeated, for the patient's "psychological defenses or confusion at some points are such that he may not hear what has been told to him." The patient is also provided some guidelines to adaptation, some guidelines to help keep him oriented during adjustment. From the topics presented earlier in this book we find Ms. Pavlou mentioning depression, anger, and communication problems between spouses as needs to be attended. "Within the group context, patients learn about available financial resources, educational and recreational opportunities, practical measures for dealing with problems from bladder control to housework."

Cammin, while discussing the Bay City, Michigan, situation, touched on the adaptive needs of the MS patients he serves. The largest group of such patients, he said "would appear to be non-neurotic individuals who are bound to have difficulty in adjusting to the very real physical, social, and economic consequences and limitations of the disease itself." It is of little value to such patients to ignore adjustments to MS, and to use "traditional approaches." In my own case it seems the physicians must even have ignored "traditional approaches," for none of them ever did anything or suggested that I do anything. Upon reflection it is easy to feel as though I had been treated like a book: once the librarian knows its contents it can be numbered and shelved; any other librarian will know something about it from the number. None of this makes any difference to the book for it is an inanimate object defined as containing the referenced information.

In closing his symposium paper, Cammin said, "It is quite often harder to adjust to the unknown than the known, and this quality of unpredictability may be an undermining factor to the patient's morale. The MS patients appear to gather considerable strength from the honest, frank exchange of information in the supportive atmosphere of our group approach." As but one married couple we agree with him and testify that the impact of our discussion group at Rush-Presbyterian-St. Luke's in Chicago is as Cammin suggests it was in Bay City.

The final topic with some commonality among the symposium papers was on personality factors. In this connection Pavlou suggested that the MS discussion group provides models which a newly diagnosed patient may need badly. Such a patient, she suggested, "is confronted with the unknown possibility of a new identity, maybe a stigmatized identity, as an MS patient." Within even a small group one can find a range of kinds of responses to difficulty, responses which sometimes reflect stable personalities, but quite often reflect unsettled, perhaps changing personalities, personalities in conflict. Some of the latter need help beyond that offered by the discussion group. Pavlou stated: "For these patients premorbid adjustment is shaky; the MS has an important meaning in terms of specific dynamic personality issues and weaknesses, and adaptive patterns are very unsatisfactory."

In Andrews' paper there were two personality themes. The first and more prominent theme suggested that personality is an influential factor in the development of the disease. Although I think one can detect a certain affinity for this theme by Andrews, she did say it "is the most controversial aspect of the MS literature."

Her second personality theme dealt with personality changes during the progress of MS. She reported a study in which MS patients were compared with patients suffering muscular dystrophy. She said that Surridge "found personality changes in both groups, but in different directions. MS patients tended to increase in both apathy and irritability, while muscular dystrophy patients tended to increase in patience and tolerance." If one is willing to incorporate irritability and apathy in a definition of personality, and if apathy can stem from fatigue or short attention span, then there is great support in this book for Surridge's findings about the alteration of the personalities of MS patients.

There was another notable feature of the symposium papers: Dr. Davis shifted from a four to a three-category characterization of MS. He retained type 1, the very mild, perhaps unsuspected and undiagnosed cases. He also retained the very severe category, which changed from type 4 to type 3. His characterization of the new type 2 encompassed both type 2 and type 3 as used throughout this book. His new type 2 is a "more moderately involved patient (with) obvious neurologic deficits, usually characterized by impairment of gait and perhaps bladder and sexual dysfunction. Some of these individuals are able to ambulate for years while others may require the use of walkers or even wheelchairs." My own preference is for the four-type analysis throughout the book.

These then are the major points from papers recently summarizing psychological research on patients with MS. Together with the review of the continuing problems of an MS patient, the papers constitute a useful base for my current consideration. Embedded in the next, and final, chapter are hints of recent work on the physical side of the condition.

Before turning to the final chapter, perhaps a nod in the direction of spouses of MS patients is due. We patients become so involved in and concerned about our condition that we overlook some of the burdens carried by our spouses.

One evening during a group meeting at the MS Center we were discussing the problems various ones of us had in connection with the operation of the sphincter valve. It was revealed that one woman stayed in the back of her house all day every day so that she would always be very near the bathroom. Her problem, of course, was the hypersensitivity which suggested to her almost constantly that she needed to urinate. It was of no avail to attempt to lead her to realize that the urge was invalid three-fourths of the time or more. The neural message is too real to the hypersensitive person to be ignored or dismissed rationally.

After a couple of such tales the husband of one patient began to tell his view of the problem. His story resonated in Kay's memory, and soon the two of them were regaling the group and chiding the patients. Kay wondered aloud how many hours she had spent waiting for me to emerge from men's rooms. She recalled that an elderly neighbor once calculated the number of days he had spent riding in the rather slow elevator in our building. It seemed to her that the number of minutes waiting for me would already sum to a number of days far surpassing that of the waiting by the lifelong elevator rider.

The husband then told of his embarrassment when

loitering in the vicinity of ladies' rooms. He felt sure that his presence was so obvious that the ladies passing by must have thought him to be at best a masher, at worst perhaps some weirdo attempting to sneak a peek as the doors swung open. Both he and Kay reported finding themselves drawn nearer the rest rooms as the minutes ticked by. Each would sometimes become concerned that their spouse was in difficulty and that they would have to arrange a rescue mission. Kay said that sometimes she thought men must have believed her to be a hooker loitering where a large volume of potential business was sure to pass.

It was clear that our spouses felt not only embarrassment, but fear and no doubt anger on occasions when the patients apparently spent undue time in the confines of rest rooms. But when hypersensitivity reads the bladder message as "now" and the sphincter valve says "not yet", and the patient is unaware of the reason for either message, undue time will be spent in rest rooms. Even knowledge of the situation does little to alleviate the frustration for the patient—or the spouse.

This recounting of events and situations by the husband of one and the wife of another patient was at times hilarious. It also served to remind the patients that it was not they alone who were affected by MS. A rejoinder to the spouses would be in order, but perhaps a joint plea by patients and spouses will help the reader understand two sources of the heavy psychological burden of multiple sclerosis.

From time to time there are references to bowel problems, including incontinence, and sexual problems, including impotence, in this book. But you will find no forthright discussion of these problems. Two reasons for this state of affairs seem valid. First, these topics are more nearly taboo in our culture than the others discussed here. Second, taboo or not, a discussion of these topics seems to reveal more about an individual than is pyschologically safe for most of us. Be assured, however, that these topics have been broached in our group discussions and it is safe to assert that bowel problems and sexual problems are on lists of difficulties characterstic of MS patients for substantial reasons.

The three discussion groups to which we have belonged have had fewer male than female MS patients. This has, perhaps, reduced the likelihood that impotence would be discussed because many times only a single male patient has been present. Since frigidity in women is a different kind of physical problem than impotence in men, a single affected male is not likely to broach the male topic in the group. But on occasions when more than one male patient has been present, the topic of impotence has been broached. The result has been that seventy-five per cent of the male patients in these groups have admitted at least temporary, occasionally sporadic, episodes of impotence. Another left the distinct impression that his wife's divorce action was heavily influenced by the fact that he had become impotent. There seemed little doubt that this male condition was a direct consequence of MS, even though one man traced his episode directly to the particular drug prescribed to alleviate a symptom of multiple sclerosis.

Incontinence was distributed across sexes in both our discussion groups and in the campers attending the MS camp the first week in September in 1974, 1975, and 1976. Both bladder and bowel were involved, occasionally in the same person. An outsized plastic, button-up, diaper-type panty is not an unknown garment among these adults, whether ambulatory or not. A well-known disposable product for babies is worn inside the plastic panty. In some cases, not ambulatory in my experience, three of the disposable pad-like products are worn. At camp we are extremely careful to guard against bed sores (they might also be termed wheelchair sores) on patients requiring such heavy protection from the consequences of incontinence. Incontinence, particularly of the bowel, traumatizes the patient absolutely. A single incident in an ambulatory patient will significantly heighten his state of tension and redirect a noticeable portion of his attention for a very long period of time, if not permanently. Make no mistake, we are now discussing fear of an intensity probably not unlike that of fear of death.

With this disturbing report we close the chapter on Current Considerations. Clearly the emphasis has been placed on psychological factors. I doubt that these factors could be overemphasized, for they are always present fueling the anxiety of both patient and spouse. The resulting behavior is often incomprehensible to the unknowing friend or observer, for many patients bear few visible symptoms of multiple sclerosis.

9
Priorities, Prognosis, and Purposes

At one point, following discovery of the uneven wearing of my shoe soles, the possibility that the cause was a minor cerebral accident, a mild stroke, occurred to me. Other events supported this belief, at least in my relative ignorance about strokes. Whether it was the areas of numbness, the partial loss of memory for words or some other symptoms I cannot now recall, but in combination with the obvious, though slight, affliction to my right leg, the symptoms suggested cerebral accident to me. Unless my physician was, and now continues withholding still more information, it seems unlikely that a stroke had occurred. At the time, of course, the fact that a diagnosis had been reached was unknown to me.

Frequent trips to the physician's office and the annual checkups, which were endured regularly, undermined confidence in my diagnosis of stroke. And so again, without knowledge of my fundamental condition and with confidence in my physician, continuing concern was my general state of mind. When one believes he is enduring symptoms of an illness or a medical condition of some kind, yet receives no such indication from a physician, one has to be concerned. If one has confidence in the physician the concern may be turned toward one's self. The resulting state can generate a more serious condition than the one being blindly endured. A fairly vivid recollection of an event at the point of my deepest depression still returns. It has been referred to earlier in this book. You may recall my words to the physician, "Go take care of your other patients; they are sick. There is nothing wrong with me." Despair had encompassed me.

Perhaps it is easy to understand what eventually drove me to seek information and advice from the staff of a research center for MS. A veritable battery of physicians, including specialists in heart, eyes, myelograms, neurology, and ears had told me nothing, or nothing which moved beyond a particular condition, moved beyond in the sense of suggesting that the condition was symptomatic of something more general and serious in nature.

With a decade and more of such treatment preceding my being informed of the diagnosis, I was ill-prepared to accept the neurologist's suggestion in 1973 that there was nothing wrong, that no symptoms were now evident. Plenty of symptoms floated to my attention from time to time, and one or two nagged continuously. I was in no position to ignore them and to stop wondering about what might occur next. The patient was at the mercy of the same sources of information about MS as were the physicians who were not specialists in MS: types of MS were not mentioned in the general literature, and, except for temporary remissions, MS was pictured as an inevitably progressive disorder.

Neither my mood nor my condition would permit me to believe that things were OK, even getting better, or perhaps just levelling off. An insistent but tricky bladder, recurring mild numbness, undeniable fatigue, continuing inability to focus attention and energy for significant periods of time, layered vision at times of eye fatigue, and hypersensitivity of the feet, all these were chronic. No use telling me otherwise; there were symptoms and I continued to be concerned. Furthermore, who could be believed? Had not a decade or more passed while games were being played with me? When finally informed of my diagnosis, I was still left to discover that my family knew. And they were left hanging, not knowing that the physician had finally informed me.

With these considerations impinging, and after many discussions with my wife, she managed successfully to urge me to contact the MS Center at Rush-Presbyterian-St. Luke's Medical Center in Chicago. That was in 1974. Few decisions have altered our life as dramatically. We were soon members of a discussion group. Discussions about the nature of MS and about particular problems stemming from the disease opened new understanding for both patient and spouse. We, Kay and I, found discussion of these matters at home were facilitated during and following the period of group sessions. Up-to-date information and theory about MS were presented by a medical research specialist in the disease. Some understanding of transpiring events as well as those past was possible because of the information presented. We began to gain some grasp of the complexity and enormity of the problems occasioned by the disease. The information provided context for our problems.

After the first couple of meetings of the discussion group, only a few weeks passed before we told our pastor of my condition. He was the first person out in the world we had faced together and informed of the situation. Next to find us capable of discussion was our daughter. For years it has been my pleasure to have luncheon with her on her birthday. We have lunched in some interesting places and in some excellent restaurants.

That particular year she and I sat high above O'Hare Airport in a revolving restaurant and discussed MS, her burdened years, and my prospects. She was eager to discuss these matters after so many years of tormented silence, and I had become a willing discussant. We idled away nearly two hours unburdening ourselves of dusty remnants from the first decade of involvement with MS, remnants no longer serving any function for us and of no particular use to anyone else. Within a few days she sent a magnificently insightful letter which I shall forever treasure.

If the experience others have had with special discussion groups focusing on MS even begins to approach that which we have had, the world should soon be abuzz with them. The advice of the first of our groups that "it's your body, seek counsel about it wherever you wish" eased the transition to medical care for MS at the center. That switch changed our lives significantly within a few hours of my first appointment. One of the most insistent and perhaps oldest of my chronic symptoms, the crotchety sphincter valve, was drugged into submission on the first try. It is necessary to remember to take some pills each day, and some moderate side effect does not escape my notice, but that valve works like a charm, allowing eight or nine hours of sleep free from its awakening and sometimes false demand for attention. Similarly, during the day there is no longer need to know the location of every restroom in town. Except for an occasional period of anxiety, such as a recent trip to Washington on behalf of the funding of a new educational program at The University of Chicago, the chemotherapy consistently works wonders on the sphincter.

When sailing became a major source of exercise, the diagnosis had not been revealed to me. Neither had drugs been suggested to control the bladder. Needless to say, I was always anxious about requiring bathroom facilities, for there were no heads on the 19-foot boats we sailed. In anticipation of a three- or four-hour lesson on the water, with a half-hour on either end when no facilities were available, I prepared all day long. A standard breakfast was followed by a light lunch with only a sip or two of water. After that there was no intake of any kind of food or beverage until the lesson was completed. This preparation enabled me to believe that the signals from the sphincter could safely be ignored for a few hours. One particular evening was difficult to manage; we were practically becalmed about a mile from our mooring, but we managed to tie up only a half-hour late. The sphincter was managed.

Just this one change, the pills, have reduced the distractions which keep energy diffused. Not that more energy is generated, for fatigue is still characteristic of my daily life, but the energy available can now be concentrated on an activity for a significant period. For example, this morning I wrote on this manuscript with riveted attention nearly an hour-and-a-half, thirty minutes past the meeting time of a committee on which I serve.

There remain symptoms of the anxiety characteristic of so many recent years of my life. For example, it is interesting to me how prone I am to seize upon any piece of information which might be related to MS, its cause, cure, or control. For example, in one issue of the *Chicago Daily News*, there was an article about the work of two researchers at The University of Chicago who are interested in diabetes. I did a "double take" while reading the following sentence: "Some results are destruction of nerve sheaths, breakdown of tiny blood vessels in the eyes and leaking of protein from blood vessels in the kidneys."

Destruction of Nerve Sheaths?! What have I been reading about? Diabetes? What else had they said? "The basic defect in diabetes," he explained, "is believed to be faulty insulin secretion by beta cells in the pancreas." And later: ". . . there is a possibility that some cases of diabetes

are caused by a virus attacking beta cells in the pancreas."
Isn't that one of the theories about MS, that a virus is involved? The researchers mention "long-time complications"
of diabetes, some of which are preventable. "Some of these
are eye damage, kidney damage, and nerve damage." I just
remembered! After suffering a couple of minor hemor-
rhages in one eye I asked our ophthalmologist about them.
She wasn't concerned, she said. Her recommendation was to
take vitamin C, which I have done religiously since then.
And then the researchers talk about "nerve damage." I
wonder . . . but it *must* be the sheath destruction that they
mentioned earlier.

The article began as follows:

> "Teaching braille to blind persons with diabetes
> was more difficult than teaching those without the
> ailment," said Dr. Arthur H. Rubenstein, University
> of Chicago Professor of medicine.

> "It was a baffling thing—until it was found that
> nerve damage caused by diabetes had impaired their
> tactile sense so they could not properly read the
> braille dots," he said.

Now the case was closing. One of the symptoms of MS
is altered tactile perception—at least altered feeling in
limbs and trunk from time to time, and weren't these attributed to damage to the nerve sheaths? The case was
nearly complete and airtight: MS is a derivative of
diabetes!

But I didn't bother to phone the investigator. This
kind of seizing on words or phrases out of context, when
features of your own illness are mentioned, is not un-
common, I suspect. Even one of the major investigations of
MS ten or fifteen years ago was apparently founded on no
more substantive base than my connection of MS and diabetes. One hopes that the association is so strong that find-

ing a preventative for diabetes will practically insure a preventative for MS. And with an article about research on
diabetes already published in a newspaper, the search for
a preventative must be nearing a successful conclusion!
How much of the time must the world move on no better
evidence or reasoning?

There is evidence that MS patients are highly susceptible to this kind of thinking, especially with regard to foods
which might prove beneficial. Elsewhere we mention caffein, linoleic acid, and bananas as being touted as exacer-
bators or inhibitors of MS. The Rush MS Center publishes
a newspaper, the *MS News,* which is "FOR People with
Multiple Sclerosis—BY People with Multiple Sclerosis."
From time to time items about foods appear. For example,
in one of the issues a patient "suggests that if you have a
problem with urinary tract infections, drink cranberry . . .
juice." In the same issue Dr. Davis says the "suggestion
concerning cranberry . . . juice is valid. Cranberry juice
tends to acidify the urine, and acidified urine is more re-
sistant to bacterial infections." This kind of comment on
"hearsay" and folk remedies helps sort the useful suggestions from the rest, and makes a valuable contribution to
the thinking of MS patients who otherwise, often in des-
peration, try dietary items which are of no value to them.
Another example of the use of the *MS News* to spread considered reports of ideas under investigation is the following
item: "Three laboratories in West Germany, England, and
Australia have separately isolated similar virus-like particles in brain tissue of MS victims. Dr. John Pinneas, University of Sidney, a researcher, also found the particles
closely associated with new damage from MS."

The *MS News* is but one example of a publication
where ideas being investigated are screened through the
consideration of thoughtful and knowledgeable people
before printing. For example, a recent annual report of the

Chicago Chapter of the National Multiple Sclerosis Society
included the following item:

> If infection by a common virus is the cause, the
> work of Dr. Hilary Koprowski and associates at the
> Wistar Institute in Philadelphia may establish the
> true cause of Multiple Sclerosis. The possibility that
> the causative factor of Multiple Sclerosis is a virus,
> does not stand in conflict with epidemiology theories,
> dealing with geographic and ethnic distribution of the
> disease.

The information getting to the public may be somewhat more valid and reliable than was the case when my
family first sought enlightenment.

A more recent issue of the *MS News*, Volume 3, No.
1, Fall–Winter, 1974, contained some very exciting information about potential help for those already stricken with
MS, the kind of information seldom found in connection
with the dread diseases.

> Starting with the experimentally established fact
> that nervous system function in multiple sclerosis is
> improved by cooling the body, Dr. Davis concluded
> that if cooling could improve nervous function effi-
> ciency, drugs might be found that would have the
> same effect but without lowering body temperature.
> Based on theoretical considerations, he used sodium
> bicarbonate injections to modify the body acid-base
> balance and oral phosphate preparations which both
> lower the blood calcium level. The experimental use
> of these drugs produce temporary improvement in
> visual functioning and they help other abnormal
> symptoms typical of multiple sclerosis. However,
> modifying the blood calcium below normal levels is
> incompatible with continued body health and such
> drugs cannot be used for other than brief experi-
> mental periods.

Such reports are heartening to all persons. Here there seems to be hope that research may help the afflicted as well as eventually controlling the causative factors of the condition.

Having attended the 1975 annual luncheon and meeting of the Chicago Chapter of the National Multiple Sclerosis Society, it seems appropriate to mention a few events which transpired there. All are related to discussions in prior chapters.

First the speaker, Dr. Foley from Cleveland, spent a noticeable segment of his time discussing urinary tract ailments among MS patients. He was, of course, referring particularly to those patients whose condition required at least occasional use of a catheter. He assured the assembly that drugs were now available to control and counteract the conditions and infections resulting from use of catheters. His feeling was that those sitting in the room and afflicted by MS might receive benefits from current research. Typically, speakers and authors suggest that current research will probably not be of benefit to those already stricken, so the idea that current patients might be helped was an exciting revelation.

Of special interest to me at the 1975 luncheon was a remark made by the very attractive young woman who at one time was the poster girl for the National Society. While she was being introduced it was noted how heavy her schedule for the day seemed to be: an early morning interview on radio, a television taping session, another live radio interview—all this before her appearance at the luncheon. Meeting this schedule was deemed a remarkable accomplishment, as indeed it was. Among her remarks was a statement that she and her companion often exercised to keep in shape for long days. She then said that they had done some yoga exercises that morning. I could not but hark back to my earlier words, "Fortunately my interest became focused on . . . exercises done by those interested in yoga." And later: "I am thankful that some methods of coping occurred naturally . . ." Here was a severely stricken patient consciously turning to the same kinds of, if not the identical, exercises to which I had been drawn unwittingly during a difficult time with a condition as yet undisclosed to me.

Before closing this chapter and the book, there is another topic to touch. It is a topic which must occur to all families in which the major provider is stricken or threatened by a serious disease. In broad terms, investigation of this topic was the second thing undertaken after being informed of the diagnosis. The topic was the probable level of financial security my wife and I would have should MS make me essentially homebound. My first reaction had been to try to determine what the diagnosis meant. Then the second step was taken and some tentative conclusions were drawn concerning financing.

First, the good news: with long-term disability insurance, disability benefits through Social Security, and some modest savings, we might survive by living modestly. Owning our home was fortunate. Payments into my retirement fund would be continued by my employer until I reached retirement age, so we could expect to enjoy the full benefits of the retirement plan.

Now the bad: if I were struck down, our present projection of funds would be frozen; that is, no salary raises would be forthcoming. Consequently, no increases in payments into retirement would be made, and no increases in retirement pay to meet inflation would be possible. With even a 2 or 3 per cent inflation gnawing away at purchasing power we would be forced to live in modest manner. Since the time of this estimate our galloping national inflation has taken wing and the previous projection has to be altered to anticipate life of a depressingly mean mode. Home ownership, as so many highly propagandized middle-class objects of value, for a year or two following our analysis and projection of life styles was turned into a projected liability. Crime rates, population movements, and hooligan activities were used as stimulants to neighborhood gossip which tended to agitate fears among older citizens and budding bigots. Home ownership amidst such activity somehow tends to lose some glamor. Consequently, projection of intentions to live where you are, for the long period probably involved were I made homebound, is difficult to generate with great confidence. To move would entail taking account of the previously mentioned rate of inflation, now applied to the real estate market.

Perhaps our economic experience has been no different from that of legions of other Americans, in the sense that our timing is poor. For example, the demand for new automobiles has always just resulted in a rise in prices when we are ready to buy. However, the bottom has always just fallen out of the used car market so that our trade-in draws less than our minimum estimate. The same bad timing would probably also affect our dealings in the real estate market. Perhaps it is clear that in the circumstances we projected, home ownership was no longer viewed as an unmixed blessing.

Obviously, perhaps, one is again forced to think seriously about priorities when projecting to years which might be spent as a homebound person. Contemplation of such a projection either forced or enabled us to set goals for points in the future, short of the time MS might strike in earnest. These goals seem useful in focusing our efforts even now that we are enjoying a period of relative stability in the course of the MS.

This particular period has also been marked by a new-found ability to inform friends of the problem. Most of our friends, of thirty years or more, know of our bout with multiple sclerosis by now. Among my physicians perhaps only the otolaryngologist remains uninformed of the diagnosis. He, no doubt, will continue to function quite well without knowing.

Perhaps by now the stated purposes for writing this book have been accomplished. If you are now more aware of the disease called multiple sclerosis, one purpose has been served. If, in addition, you are more knowledgeable about the patterns of symptoms which emanate from the several (multiple) minute patches of scar tissue (sclerosis) which replace the destroyed myelin covering of the nerves, then the second purpose has been served. A third purpose, to proclaim that the effect of having MS, whether revealed to the patient or not, is staggering in the psychological mode, has been accomplished. My hope is that many physicians will soon be brought to realize that what is proclaimed here is also true.

Paradoxically, perhaps, some physicians disregard, even deny the physical symptoms and with careless arrogance suggest that the problem is psychological. A new friend, whom we have known for a year, is one of those persons who has arisen from the MS bed and returned to a rather full, ambulatory life. But it is not about her recovery that I report. Rather, it is to incorporate her experience with physicians with regard to the diagnosis of MS. She says that her physician kept telling her, in the early days of her symptoms, that "It is all in your head." If so, she certainly willed herself into a condition with symptoms bearing a remarkable resemblance to MS. As she reports about her acquaintances who have had the same experience, that is being told, "It is all in your head," her disgust with physicians in general is obvious.

Perhaps it is time to lay the pencil aside. Having entered a period of remission, with a principal chronic complaint under the control of a drug and the mildly recurring symptoms somewhat better understood, speculation about the future course of my MS is guarded. My full energy capacity has not returned, nor has my ability to concentrate attention and focus energy in an intense and sustained fashion. However, some progress seems noticeable in these problem areas. Some of my leg muscles are losing strength. This is particularly noticeable in attempts to help carry someone up a few steps. If my position in lifting necessitates moving backward up the steps, there is no hope. I am completely unable to do this chore, standing as if frozen into position. This particular weakening is evident from year to year in helping campers at the annual MS camp. It may reflect my advancing age, but I exercise diligently each morning and have for many years in an effort to stave off this very problem of weakening legs. Other persistent, though manageable symptoms have been mentioned earlier in this chapter.

Undoubtedly, I hope we are better prepared to deal with the future than we were when Kay, Diane and I struggled, each alone and in different swamps of ignorance and misinformation, better even than when we wrestled with the known diagnosis but without useful insight into the condition. Clearly there are symptoms with which you must live throughout the remainder of life, whether yours is type 2, 3, or 4 MS. We are learning to adapt to my type 2, sometimes 2½, symptoms as a result of learning more about the basic condition. But before finally ending this tale about MS, let me mention one last experience.

Kay and I attended the Chicago MS Chapter's MS camp as volunteers in 1974, 1975, and 1976. It was more than an interesting experience, more nearly a revelation. A wide range of disabling conditions were represented among the campers, although in the main they had MS. Except for a minor, limited incident or two the campers thoroughly enjoyed themselves. They rode trails through the woodlands in a large covered trailer pulled behind a tractor. This trailer held perhaps ten wheelchairs, with squeeze-in room along the sides for mobile campers and some staff who accompanied each trip. Swimming in a beautiful, specially equipped, heated, outdoor pool was an enjoyable time for all. Some campers could swim a little, others could float. An occasional camper learned to swim. Some enjoyed being propelled about by staff members who also encouraged movement of seldom-used limbs and muscles. It was a toss-up between the overnight campout and square dancing in wheelchairs as to which engendered the more riotous enjoyment.

The activities were taken over by the campers at meal times when "lost" items could be reclaimed only after performance of a song, poem or story. On stunt night, after games were played, some of the marvelous musical talent among the campers was displayed for the enjoyment of all. Each camper had an opportunity to blossom as a unique individual and most did if only for a few fleeting moments.

At camp everybody was in a similar boat, so to speak, and the staff was largely volunteer, so problems which might have been upsetting for someone at home were hardly noticeable, routine affairs in the camp setting. A call for assistance in the middle of the night seemed to waken only staff members, who were always ready to serve. A change of bed linens and a shower were available around the clock. The facilities were designed for the use of crippled children and so presented ramps, wide doors, wide bathroom stalls with railings and bars on the walls, a shower room with a relatively dry central area and moveable chairs for those who could not stand to shower, and many other well-planned features. The sinks had been designed to accommodate shavers in wheelchairs. Those responsible for making decisions about public facilities for handicapped persons would benefit from a visit to this camp or another facility like it. They would quickly realize the many barriers which handicapped persons face in simply going to a store.

Recollection of the camp experience brings with it another topic which has been touched upon previously: food, or perhaps nutrition is the proper word. At camp in 1974 there were bananas available for at least two meals a day. Even more striking to Kay and me was that no one ever mentioned this fact. Certainly the appearance of so many bananas at any other camp we have attended would have triggered a variety of comments, but not so at the MS camp. We recalled having read that potassium is lacking in MS patients and that bananas are an excellent source. I recall beginning to purchase and consume bananas almost daily. Three years later we still have a banana with breakfast. It was evident at camp that others had heard the word too, and bananas were as much a part of the camp as trail-rides. The supply of bananas has been reduced in subsequent years at camp, but they have not disappeared.

Endless tales of fun at camp could be told. And some heart-rending stories are at hand. But I should like to close in a personal vein because my situation is well known to me. I suspect, however, that the ambivalence I feel about my condition is reflective of the attitude of many thousands whose condition is very similar.

As has been said before, many symptoms persist or recur too regularly for me to be mindless of multiple sclerosis. However, the disease seems to be in remission, in the sense that new symptoms have not appeared for months. We hope that the remission is permanent, that the MS has "burned out."

Even if it has run its course there remain two kinds of residuals: the scarred nerve coverings may always remain to float up an old symptom of one kind of another. Thus, for example, if someone asks whether my eyes are

OK I must say that in general they are, but layered vision still appears at times. Finally, MS struck me at the tag end of the age of susceptibility, and the potentially productive decade-and-a-half beginning with age 36 was dissipated struggling with the condition rather than developing in my career line. This second residual seems the more difficult to live with, for there is never a period of remission to be anticipated or enjoyed.

But believe me, this fate is easier to handle than another from which I may have been saved. Furthermore, it has been an interesting condition to encounter and contemplate. Let us hope that in the near future others may be denied the privilege of contemplation of a personal encounter with MS.

Index

Abdomen, 39–41, 53, 77
Acta Neurologica Scandinavia, 121
ACTH, 119
Adaptive needs, 122, 126
Adjustment, 96, 119, 123, 126, 127. *See also* Psychological adjustment
Aggression, 78, 82–83, 92, 96, 116
Altered sensation, 44, 49, 106, 138. *See also* Hypersensitivity; Numbness
American Psychological Association (APA), Symposium, viii, 45, 96, 117, 119, 121–22, 126
Andrews, Susan L., viii, 45, 96, 123–24, 128
Anesthetic, 37–38
Anger, 31, 123, 126
Antibodies, 18
Anxiety, 114

Arthritis, 89–90
Ataxia, 23, 78, 119
Attention: focusing, 47–49, 58, 78, 85–86, 107, 132, 135; span of, 46–47, 85, 128
Autoimmune mechanism, 16–18, 89

Balance, 9, 66
Bay City, Michigan, 126
Belfast, 125
Billings Hospital, 59; library, 11–12
Bladder, 10, 18, 24, 62–63, 70, 76, 78, 85, 100, 126, 130–31, 134. *See also* Incontinence
Blindness. *See* Vision
Blood: analysis, 125; donor, 35; flow, 15; transfusion, 33; white cells, 125
Bowel problems, 18, 130–31. *See also* Incontinence
Brain: damage, 124–26;